the nude
nutritionist

To be honest and 'stripped bare', as my TV name suggests, no images of me have been photoshopped for this book – or anywhere else! When we're constantly seeing photographs that have been retouched, filtered and only depict one image of health and beauty, it's so easy to forget that no 'body' is perfect. Health truly comes in different shapes, colours and sizes. It's hard enough to love your body in a society that tells you not to, and that's why I'm committed to always keeping it real and being photoshop-free.

the nude nutritionist

STOP OBSESSING ABOUT FOOD + NEVER DIET AGAIN

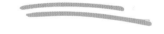

Lyndi Cohen

MURDOCH BOOKS
SYDNEY · LONDON

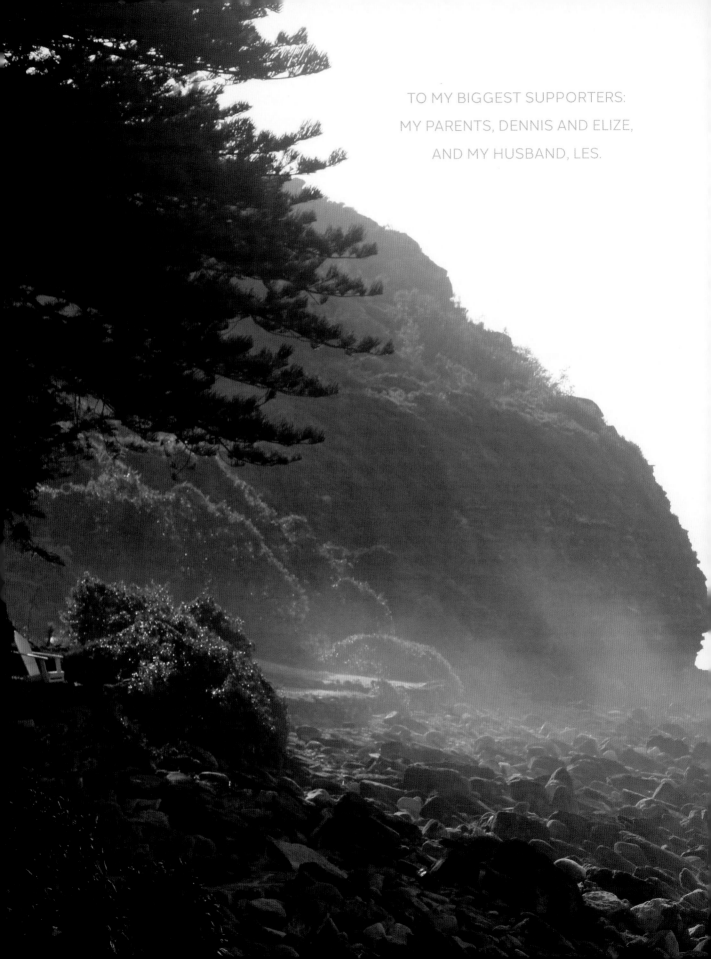

TO MY BIGGEST SUPPORTERS:
MY PARENTS, DENNIS AND ELIZE,
AND MY HUSBAND, LES.

Contents

My story · 7

1 How to spot a diet in disguise · 13

2 Become an intuitive eater · 19

3 Stripped back to basics · 33

4 How to keep it real · 55

5 Heal your relationship with food · 77

6 Boost your body image · 99

7 Feel amazing · 117

Recipes · 141

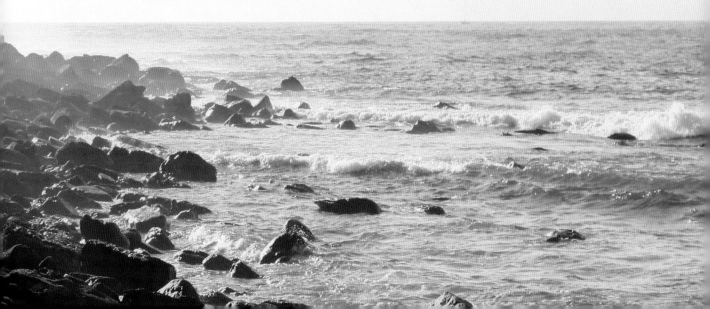

My story

No-one ever intends to binge eat, but depriving yourself isn't sustainable. You might be happy to starve into a version of yourself that you like, but I know from experience that your body has other plans. This book is about learning to eat healthily without obsessing, so you can go to bed at night feeling comfortable in your own skin and at peace.

When I was growing up, I was dedicated to losing weight the way some people are dedicated to winning gold at the Olympic Games. I wasn't passionate about nutrition so much as obsessed with losing weight. I was bigger than most other girls my age, something I first realised when I was six years old while wearing my too-tight pink leotard in ballet class. I remember comparing the other girls' bodies to mine. My legs were thicker, my tummy was naturally more rounded and my frame was definitely bigger. I was self-conscious about my body, but my size didn't seem to be a real problem for me until I hit puberty.

While my weight was within a healthy range, I started to care more about what I looked like and thought I needed to be slim to be liked. This triggered my obsession with losing weight. I saw my first nutritionist and she seemed nice, but it was clear from our first session that if I wanted to be 'slim' (and everything around me told me that I did), I was no longer allowed to eat the same foods that my brothers ate. From then on, I had special low-calorie diet snacks and meals in small portion sizes. I watched in envy while my twin older brothers ate what they wanted. I was 11 years old.

As I grew older, it turned out that I was willing to sacrifice a lot to try to lose weight. Counting calories and 'trying to be good' was my life's mission. I'd lie in bed scrutinising what I'd eaten that day and swearing that I'd be better tomorrow. I started avoiding social occasions that involved food and created a

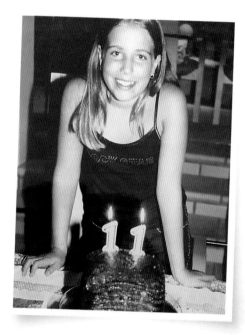

This is me aged 11, when my obsession with dieting began.

long list of 'bad' or forbidden foods. Food was constantly on my mind.

Diet and exercise

I always had a goal weight; a magic number that I hoped one day to weigh. I imagined that when I reached this goal, I would finally love my body and be proud of myself. So I tried all the well-known diets; I did programs that promised body transformation within weeks and endured gruelling boot camps. I googled articles about losing weight and I bought every women's magazine that claimed it could teach you how to look like the photoshopped model on the front cover.

But even once I got to my goal weight, it never felt the way I imagined. I'd still look at photos of myself and think: 'Your arms are still so big. You could still lose more weight.' And so the goalposts kept moving.

Weigh-ins would happen first thing in the morning, before having anything to eat or drink. I'd strip off my clothes and stare at myself in the full-length mirror. I'd make sure the scale was in the right place then step on, nervous and excited. Some mornings, the scale gave me the answer I wanted. I had lost weight. But the relief was only short-lived.

As time went on, I became more disordered in my relationship with food and the scales. I'm ashamed to admit it, but one night before a morning weigh-in with a dietitian I cut my hair into a bob in an attempt to weigh less at the appointment. I was left with a lopsided hairdo and a heavy sense of shame. I left her office sobbing, devastated by being such a failure. I was 15 years old.

Eventually, even when I ate 'well' all week, I wouldn't lose weight. The scales went from being a friendly motivator to cruel enemy.

After years of letting myself go hungry, my metabolism had slowed as my body no longer trusted me to feed it properly. To protect me (and because my body loved me even when I didn't love it) my body held onto the weight.

My willpower was depleted. It didn't take me long to say, 'Screw it! I've messed up today already. I may as well finish this. I'll just start again tomorrow.'

Bingeing and emotional eating

I'd wait till the house was empty. Even then, I would hide in the pantry and gorge myself on all the 'bad' foods I wasn't 'allowed' to eat. I'd sneak food to my bedroom and then hide the wrappers. I'd sometimes replace food to cover up my shameful secret. I was so ashamed.

Typically, I would only stop eating when someone came home, or I ran out of food, or I was just too tired to continue. I'd go to sleep hating and reprimanding myself for another failed day. Then I would wake up in the morning and try to be 'good' to undo all the 'bad' food I had eaten. By the afternoon, I was ravenous and deprived. A binge was inevitable and I stayed stuck in the emotional eating cycle.

In my mind, I wasn't 'on a diet' because I hadn't bought a specific book or subscribed to

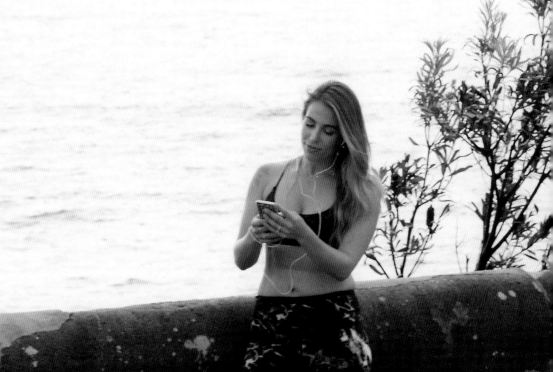

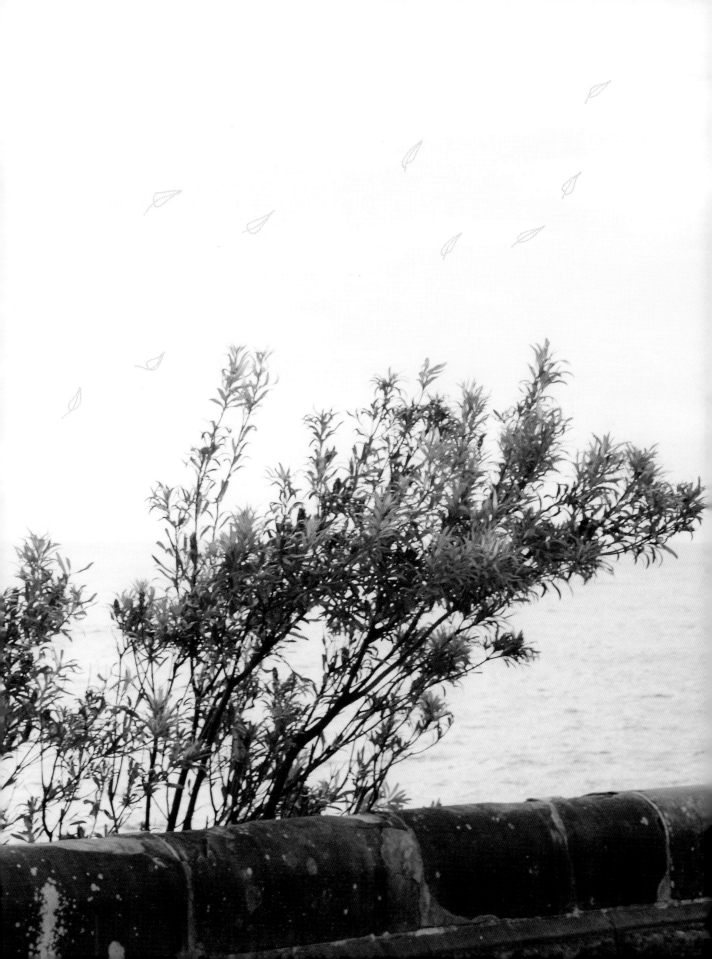

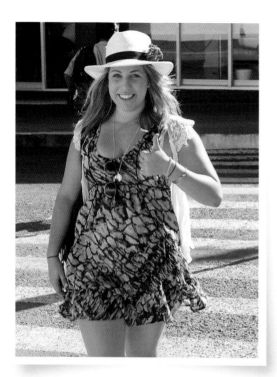

This photo was taken a decade after I started dieting, when I was 21 years old.

a certain program; but I was controlled by my own set of rules that I had adopted over years of having an obsession with losing weight.

A change of attitude

My breaking point came in 2011, when I received a diagnosis that rocked me to my core. Being told I had clinical anxiety came as a big shock. When I left the doctor's office, I cried. I had known for a while that I was not winning: my turbulent relationship with food, my poor body image and the constant blows to my self-confidence were feeding the anxiety.

The decision to stop trying to control everything I ate was really scary. Gaining weight was my biggest fear, but I realised that years of dieting had made me hate my body and gain weight. Slowly, I adopted an intuitive approach to food, that didn't involve calorie counting, deprivation, punishment or cutting out foods. I stopped weighing myself and bought clothing that actually fitted me. Instead of ignoring my body cues, I began

listening to my hunger. My main objective became about being healthy, not skinny. I started doing the things you'll learn about in this book.

This wasn't a swift or easy process. I was still desperate to lose weight and it was so tempting to go on another diet. Every day I needed to reassure myself that I was doing the right thing. Every meal would push me outside my comfort zone. I decided that going to bed feeling at peace with myself was more important than the number on the scale. And then the weight started to come off. Within four years, I had lost more than 20 kg (44 lb). But do you know what? The weight loss turned out to be just an added bonus.

The real victory was that my life wasn't controlled by food any more. For the first time in my adult life, I had so much more time and headspace to think about more important things. I began to eat to feel healthy and energised and I exercised, not to punish myself for eating, but because I enjoyed it. Best of all, I stopped needing to console myself with food.

So that was the start of my journey and I bet you can relate to the way I felt and the way I acted. In this book, I am going to share with you the things I did to stop dieting, end emotional eating and regain control over my attitude to food. I'll also help you find balance with your mood and hormones so you can feel lighter, more energetic and finally feel comfortable in your body. I am going to teach you a refreshingly different approach that will help you live healthily, without constantly thinking about food. And that's just the start.

If you're sick of constantly dieting and hating your body, then it's time to learn a new approach. Healthy eating isn't meant to be hard: and I'm proof that it's not. So come along and I'll show you how!

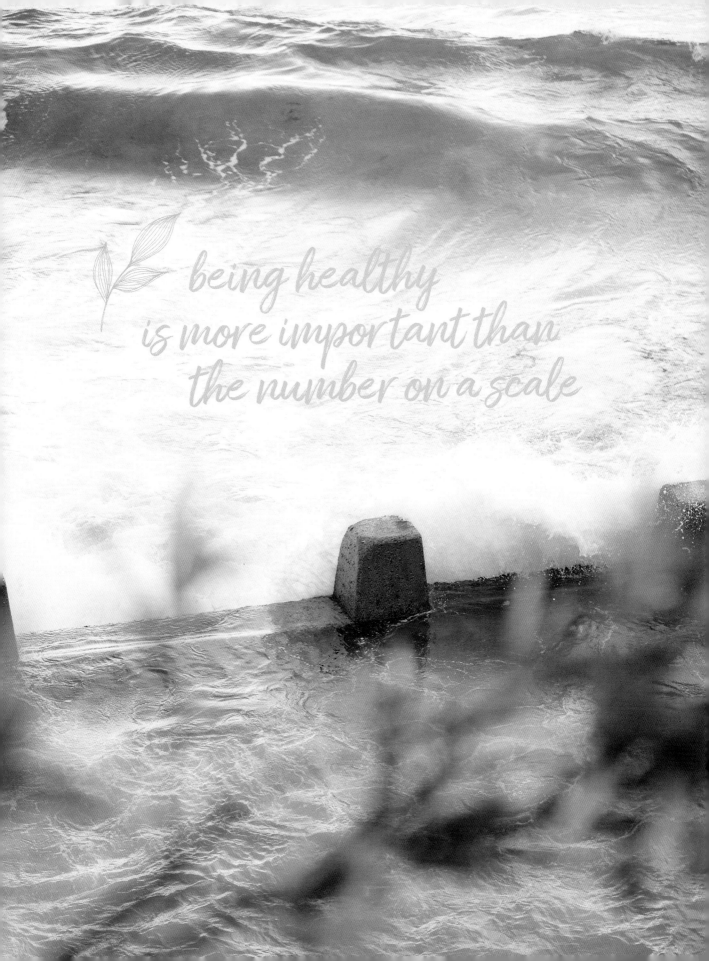

being healthy
is more important than
the number on a scale

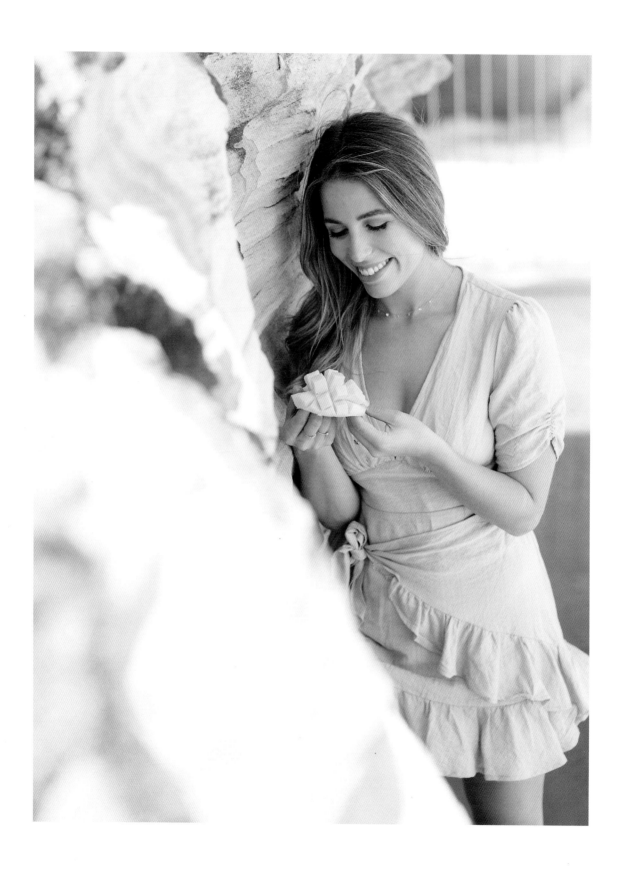

1

How to spot a diet in disguise

Diets suck. They suck the joy out of healthy eating and the soul from your social life. Any weight loss and health gains tend to last about as long as a celebrity marriage, leaving you with yet another failure. Giving up dieting is the best thing I ever did; and the first step to quitting dieting is to learn how to spot a diet in disguise.

I bet you already know that diets don't work in the long term. And yet I can almost guarantee that you're on a diet right now and you don't even realise it.

Don't worry: most people diet by mistake. Every day, I meet crazy-smart-funny-talented people who are on a diet and don't know it. Traditional diets are easy to spot; the word 'diet' is often in the name, which is a dead giveaway. Gotcha! These diets come with a set of rules and a meal plan to follow and if you don't pay for the plan you are usually expected to buy foods and supplements to help you along the way.

Yet most diets aren't as dizzyingly obvious as this and, unfortunately, the most damaging diet is the diet in disguise. These days many diets are 'undercover'. Marketers and social-media starlets got the hint that diets were out and 'balance' was cool. To capitalise on this new approach, they hype their highly profitable books and programs as 'a fad-free balanced approach to nutrition without diets', but read on and you'll soon be told to cut out gluten, alcohol, sugar, wheat or fruit. This, my friends, is a diet in disguise and they're the worst. Diets are often well-camouflaged as 'healthy eating' but take note when you see words such as: foods to avoid, clean eating, detox, grain-free, sugar-free, superfoods and toxic. These are clues that you may be looking at a diet in disguise.

For 10 years I dieted by mistake, and it kept me struggling with my weight and caught in the vicious emotional-eating cycle. If you'd asked, I would have told you confidently that diets don't work and that I was simply 'eating healthily' or 'trying to be good'.

What I didn't realise is that I was controlled by dieting rules. For as long as I believed that I shouldn't have carbs after 5 pm, that I should eat six small meals a day or that breakfast is the most important meal of the day, I was on a diet and would continue to struggle with my weight. I truly believed the rules kept my weight down and I feared that if I stopped following these rules, my weight would spiral further out of control.

I was wrong. Once I stopped trying to control food, food stopped controlling me. And it was so liberating. Dieting rules, not my willpower, had been the problem the whole time. Diet rules made me fear perfectly nutritious food, made me obsessed with health and left me feeling guilty when I deviated even slightly from 'the plan'.

Dieting (by mistake) was the reason I was out of control around food and was struggling with my weight. A lot of recent research has shown that dieting leads to weight gain in the long term. This is because restrictive diets:

- Slow your metabolism
- Make you feel deprived
- Increase cravings for 'forbidden foods'
- Cause you to obsess about food or think about food all the time
- Trigger binge and emotional eating
- Set you up for a disordered relationship with food

The truth is that all diets work. The question is: do you want to live on that diet for the rest of your life? If you don't want to fast for two days

DO YOU WANT TO BE *on a diet* YOUR ENTIRE LIFE?

Tip

Quitting sugar, avoiding gluten and 'clean eating' are often diets in disguise.

of your week or avoid your favourite foods for the rest of your life, then there isn't any point doing it for a few weeks because you'll quickly regain any weight you lose—plus more!—when the diet inevitably ends.

It's thought that as many as 95 per cent of diets fail in the longer term. That's seriously terrible odds! It's like a parachute that fails to open 95 out of 100 times. If you were one of the lucky people who survived, you'd be celebrated in the media for beating the odds. And this is exactly what we do when people successfully lose weight on a diet. Their stories are splashed across news sites and magazines. As a result, you come to believe that every day, people just like you are having success with diets. This reporting bias causes you to overestimate how successful you'll be on a diet and tricks you into thinking that 'THIS diet is different and it will work'. But it's all a trick.

So you try yet another diet. At the start, your motivation is high but soon you hit a roadblock—you don't lose weight as quickly as you thought you would, you miss going out for drinks with your friends, you get too busy at work to exercise, meal prep begins to feel too

hard—and your motivation starts to dwindle. With each new diet attempt, your ability to sustain motivation gets smaller. That's because each time you try to lose weight on a diet, it's harder and harder. The weight is more stubborn; your body is more reluctant to let the fat go; and your willpower diminishes with each new attempt.

So instead of losing weight and keeping it off, each time you try another diet, you end up losing willpower, and then you regain more weight than you lost in the first place. Over time, your relationship with food gets worse and worse, and your weight goes up and up.

It's not your fault. Diets set you up for failure. The good news is that once you become aware of diets in disguise and decide you're ready to live a truly diet-free life, without restriction, counting calories or clean eating, you can learn how to keep it real, stop obsessing and never be a victim of diets again. The first step is to ditch those pesky dieting rules that keep you stuck in the emotional-eating, food-guilt and body-hate cycle. To do this, you need to become aware of all the food rules you currently subscribe to.

DIETING GETS IN THE WAY OF:

- Leading a healthy life
- Reducing emotional eating
- Feeling in control of your body
- Trusting your body
- Feeling calm around food
- Accepting and loving your body
- Reaching your healthiest weight

WHEN YOU DIET, YOU DON'T CONTROL FOOD
food controls you

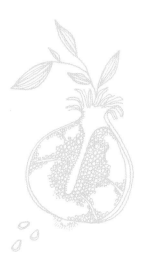

Are you on a diet in disguise?

You might not be aware of the extent to which your eating is dictated by dieting rules. Try this simple exercise: photocopy the worksheet on the facing page and fill in the answers, then consider the following questions.

For each diet rule you ticked, ask yourself:

- Do I feel guilty when I don't do this behaviour?
- When I break this diet rule, do I feel bad about myself or feel guilty?
- Does this behaviour cause me to think about food more? Does it make me feel obsessed with food?

If the answer to any of these questions is yes, then this diet rule is most certainly a diet in disguise.

Like getting over an ex, the less time you spend thinking about it, the easier it is. Dieting rules often make you think about food more, which does not help you eat less or more nutritiously.

From now on, notice when you start to ask yourself: 'Am I allowed to eat this?' Asking this questions is a symptom of being stuck in the diet mentality. Because of course you're allowed to eat it. The more important question is: do you want to eat it? How will eating it make you feel? Food must be a choice, not feel like a prison sentence.

Changing the question to, 'I am allowed to eat that, but do I really want to?' is the key. The distinctions are subtle, but can make an oh-so-significant difference.

Are you dieting by mistake?

Is your 'healthy lifestyle' just a diet in disguise?
Use this checklist to identify your diet rules.

√ *Tick all that apply*

☐ Don't have carbs after lunch

☐ Breakfast is the most important meal of the day

☐ Eat six small meals a day to keep my metabolism going

☐ Have protein at every meal

☐ Chew gum, or drink water or diet soft drinks when hungry

☐ Eat at the same time every day

☐ Order salad dressing on the side

☐ Don't eat after 8 pm at night

☐ Other _____

You might also say, 'I'm not dieting, I'm just...'

☐ Trying to be 'good'

☐ Following a meal plan

☐ Avoiding gluten (even though I'm not coeliac or sensitive)

☐ Cutting out all sugar or foods containing sugar

☐ Cutting out all junk food

☐ Avoiding alcohol to lose weight

☐ Eating 'clean'

☐ Doing a cleanse

☐ Cutting out wheat/dairy/meat/carbs/other in order to lose weight

☐ Weighing myself daily or weekly

☐ Saying no to social occasions so I can eat more healthily

☐ Detoxing

☐ Tracking what I eat with a calorie counter

☐ Trying not to binge

☐ Limiting treats to a 'cheat meal'

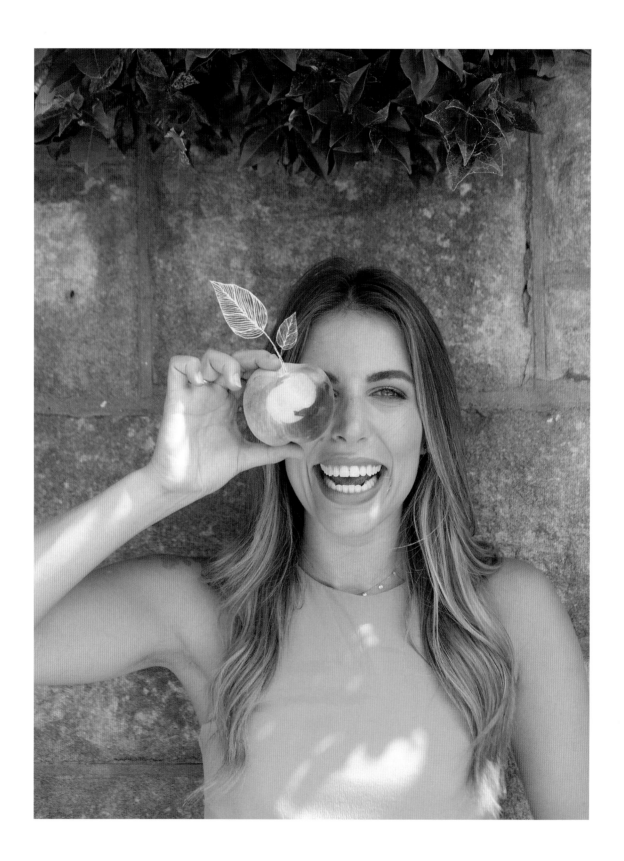

2

Become an intuitive eater and stop dieting *for good*

Intuitive eating is a simple way of reconnecting with your body and food, so that eating becomes easy and, well, intuitive! It's the exact opposite of dieting (so you know it's got to be good for you). I certainly didn't come up with the idea of intuitive eating, but learning how to do it changed my life.

Now that you know how to spot a diet (even one in disguise), you're ready to learn more about intuitive eating. Luckily, intuitive eating doesn't require following any rules and you don't need any special equipment. In fact, you can start doing it right now. Hooray!

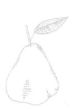

Are you ready to stop dieting, struggling with your weight and obsessing over everything you eat? I'm excited for you, because I remember exactly where I was when I first learned about intuitive eating: the concept immediately made sense to me. Why had I never heard about this before? As soon as I understood the principles of intuitive eating, I knew it would change my life. This is what I learned.

From the moment you were born, you intuitively knew how much food your body needed to get enough energy. You cried when you were hungry and stopped eating when you were satisfied. You did not need a meal plan to tell you the best way to eat for your blood type or a diet book to guide your eating. You were born understanding how to best fuel your body so that you thrived, grew strong and healthy; however, as you grew older, all of this changed.

As a toddler, your eating schedule was carved out based on meal times, your sleep patterns and your parents' needs. As a child, well-intentioned advice—for example, 'finish everything on your plate'—dulled your intuitive eating skills further, so you learned to eat even when you weren't hungry. When you were well behaved you were rewarded with treats and you were denied dessert if you misbehaved.

As you grew into a teenager, diet rules—for example, 'eat six small meals a day to keep your metabolism going' and 'avoid carbohydrates and fat to lose weight'—made intuitive eating near impossible. And it's around that time that you probably began to eat when you were bored, tired or stressed out.

Soon, everyone was giving you nutrition advice on the best way to eat: the latest celebrity, your mum, your best friend, the personal trainer at the gym, your neighbour and the hairdresser. Instead of listening to your own body and eating when you were hungry, you turned to others to guide you. Unfortunately, no-one other than you can truly know the best way to fuel your body. You are so unique and you are the expert on your body.

Intuitive eating is about turning away from the confusing (and often contradictory) diet rules, the noise and nonsense and getting back that very deeply intelligent part of you that knows exactly how best to feed yourself. When you eat intuitively, your body will help you naturally regulate your weight and help you choose the right amount of food you need to thrive and feel amazing. You don't need a meal plan or a diet guru to tell you how or what to eat, all you have to do is check in with your hunger and how your food makes you feel.

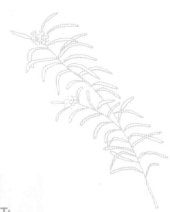

Intuitive eating

The best indicator of how much energy your body needs is your appetite. If you 'eat by the clock' (that is, you eat breakfast because it's breakfast time) or follow a meal plan, you tend to ignore your appetite and eat because you think you should. But are you even hungry most of the time when you eat?

Your appetite is a primal system that is designed to ensure you get enough energy to fuel your body and to regulate your weight, preventing you from losing or gaining too much. That's right! You were born with your own built-in weight-management system.

Tuning into your appetite

On days when your body needs more energy, you will feel more hungry. When you don't need as much energy, your appetite will be smaller. When you listen and respond to your appetite, you are able to fuel your body with the ideal amount of energy it needs. No calorie counter needed, just your own innate intelligence.

Your body will also help you work out which foods are better for you by providing valuable feedback. Chances are you feel energetic, healthy and amazing when you eat foods such as a home-cooked meal or salad, but feel bloated, tired and heavy after eating processed fast-food meals. When you listen and respond to your body, you end up naturally craving more nutritious options because it makes you feel good, not because you think you should.

WHEN YOU STOP AND LISTEN TO YOUR BODY, YOU MIGHT NOTICE THAT:

- You often eat because you think you should, out of habit or when you're bored. You often aren't as hungry as you thought you were.
- Some weeks you are naturally hungrier than others, and need more food. Some days, your appetite is less intense and you're happy to enjoy lighter options.
- Your body really does know the best time for you to eat.

There is no meal plan that can meet your body's constantly changing needs throughout the day, week, month or year. Intuitive eating simplifies eating so you no longer have to ask: 'Should I eat this? Am I allowed to eat this?' (Very confusing questions!)

Instead, you can simply ask: 'Am I hungry? Will this food make me feel good?' To answer, you only need to consult yourself, the expert on your body.

You'll be surprised how simply becoming aware of your hunger and appetite in the first instance can help change your thinking and relationship with food.

Are you excited? I hope so because I'm about to introduce you to the hunger scale, an incredibly simple tool that can help you become a more intuitive eater.

Hunger scale

TOO HUNGRY	*0*	Beyond hungry. Empty stomach.
	1	Ravenous. Weak and dizzy.
HUNGRY	*2*	Very hungry. Irritable. Low energy.
	3	Comfortably hungry. Ideal time to eat something.
	4	Peckish. Getting hungry. Feel like 'I could eat'.
NEUTRAL	*5*	Neutral. Neither hungry nor full.
	6	Slighty full or getting full.
FULL	*7*	Comfortably full. Ideal time to stop eating.
	8	Quite full.
TOO FULL	*9*	Very full. Uncomfortable.
	10	Stuffed. Too full. Feel sick.

The hunger scale

The hunger scale is a simple tool that can help you work out just how hungry you are. Ranking your hunger, on a scale from 0–10, can help you better respond to your appetite and be an intuitive eater.

Using the hunger scale is easy. Before you eat, rank your hunger on a scale of zero to 10. Zero is beyond hungry and 10 is stuffed full. It can help to think of the hunger scale like the fuel gauge for your car. The fuel light is your hunger, reminding you to top up on some food. It may take about 30 minutes to move one point along the hunger scale. So if you're neutral (5), you may be hungry (3) in an hour.

> ** Hangry: When you're so hungry you become angry (0–2 on the hunger scale).*

If you ignore the fuel light, you might run out of energy and become a zero or one on the hunger scale. At this point, you're in dangerous territory! You're so low on energy that you'll struggle to make rational decisions and might feel dizzy, light-headed, moody or 'hangry'.* When you are ravenous, your body is desperate to fill your tank (stomach) with energy in the quickest and easiest way possible. This is why you'll often reach for convenient, carbohydrate-based comfort foods, such as bread, cereal, chips, cake, lollies (candy or sweets) and more. In this primal state, your body demands food that will give you a big hit of calories, real fast.

When you're ravenous, it doesn't matter what good intentions you have, your body has flipped into a primal fight-or-flight mode and will do anything to ensure its basic need for fuel is met. This is why you shouldn't go

become an intuitive eater ∿∿∿

grocery shopping or arrive at a party ravenous. Many people who 'try to be good' to lose weight (diet in disguise), allow themselves to get overly hungry. The result is almost always the same. They end up eating everything in sight, then feel guilty and ashamed instead of recognising that they were simply too hungry to be in control. By using the hunger scale to assess your appetite, you can prevent yourself from getting too hungry, helping you to feel more in control around food.

When you wait too long to eat and you're ravenous (0–1 on the hunger scale), you also end up eating very fast, without really tasting or enjoying your food. You often keep eating until you are past satisfied and eat until you feel stuffed or bloated (9–10 on the hunger scale). Like being too hungry, being too full doesn't feel good either.

When you eat too much and feel stuffed, you may feel sick, get stomach cramps, grow tired and feel irritable. And each time you overeat, your stomach becomes a little more stretched. Eventually, this makes you hungrier and means you have more stomach to fill each time you eat.

As you begin to eat food, your stomach sends hormones (chemical messengers) to your brain to switch off hunger and make you feel full and satiated. This process can take 10–30 minutes, which is why it's important to eat slowly and not be distracted. If you are distracted and ignore your body when it tells you that it's satisfied, your stomach will continue to stretch beyond its normal limits, causing discomfort when you become overly full (9–10 on the hunger scale). If you regularly overeat, your stomach capacity increases. As a result, you need more food to fill your stomach before you feel full. You might also become resistant to leptin, the hormone that makes you feel satisfied, and more sensitive to hunger hormones. You can easily understand that this is how your weight can 'spiral out of control'.

YOU EAT BEFORE YOU GET HUNGRY BECAUSE:

- It's 'mealtime' (breakfast, lunch, dinner). This is known as 'eating by the clock'.
- You're bored
- You're happy or celebrating with food
- Something stressful happens
- You pre-emptively eat before you're hungry, in case you get hungry later.
- Something tastes really good!
- You feel peckish

The good news is that when you tune into your natural hunger cues and stop dieting, you reduce out-of-control eating. Your stomach will shrink again and you'll naturally feel more satiated from eating less. You'll also get fuller quicker, and find it easier to stop eating once you've had enough. As you learn how to keep it real, you'll trust that you can always have more if you want!

When is the ideal time to eat?

Ideally, your hunger should always range between three and seven on the hunger scale. Imagine your hunger is like a pendulum that swings from side to side. You want to avoid swinging to the extremes on either side of the hunger scale: too hungry (0–1) and too full (9–10). But you also don't want to eat before you get hungry!

It's important to wait until you become hungry before you eat. When you eat when you're neutral (5 on the hunger scale), instead

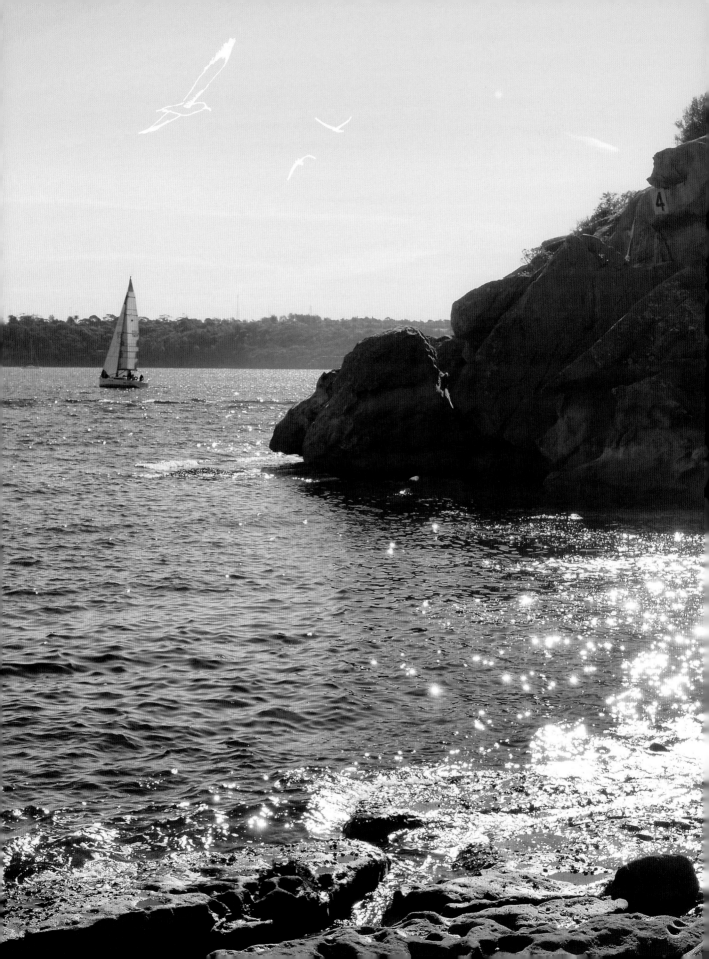

If you're scared of getting caught without food, keep a couple of pieces of fruit in your handbag or a handful of nuts in a handy container. That way you can practise listening to your hunger without fear that you'll become ravenous because you've got nothing to eat.

of waiting until you are hungry (3 on the hunger scale), you're jumping the gun! You don't go and sit on the toilet when you don't need to go, so there is no need to eat when you aren't hungry. Hunger is your body's way of saying, 'I'd love more energy soon as I've run out of available energy supply. Please top me up with energy.'

In the developed world, we get anxious and scared about feeling even slightly hungry. Diets promise that you'll lose weight and 'never feel hungry'. We have been taught to fear hunger, especially if we were raised by parents who grew up without ready access to food, but when you have abundant access to food, feeling comfortably hungry is OK. Not only does food taste much better when you are hungry, but feeling comfortably hungry is healthy, as long as you don't get too hungry!

Sometimes, you will eat when you aren't hungry—for example, you have a piece of cake at a party—and that is OK! Wait to feel hungry before eating most of the time, but leave some wriggle room for living in the moment, being flexible and enjoying life.

Ideally, you want to stop eating when you feel satisfied. Stopping before you get too full is easier said than done and you may not get it right every time. As you practise listening to your hunger, stopping when you reach 7 on the hunger scale will become easier and you'll be less likely to keep overeating. Occasionally, you may still eat more than you want (until you are overfull) or when you aren't hungry, but

that is normal and human. It'll happen! Over time, you'll come to trust that any time you need more food, you're allowed to eat it.

After years and years of dieting, it can be tricky to work out how hungry you are. Because you've been programmed to ignore your hunger and follow diet rules, this is totally normal. With practice, you will get better at waiting to feel hungry before eating and finishing your meal when you feel satiated. Here are some strategies to help.

EAT WHEN YOU FEEL HUNGRY
(3 on the hunger scale)

FINISH EATING WHEN YOU FEEL SATISFIED
(7 on the hunger scale)

Could you wait any longer?
Once you know that you're physically hungry, ask yourself, 'could I wait 30 minutes before eating or will I be too hungry by then?' Sometimes, you can wait. Sometimes, you really can't wait and need food now! Although each of us is different, it often takes around 30–45 minutes to move one point along the hunger scale, in either direction. If you're at neutral (5) now, it might take an hour to an

hour and a half to become hungry (3). Start tuning in to your appetite and learn how long it takes you to reach the next stage.

It's OK to leave food on your plate

Did you grow up being instructed to finish everything on your plate? This becomes a habit that forces you to keep eating even when you feel satisfied. To help break this habit, you may want to practise leaving a mouthful of food on your plate when you finish eating, provided you feel full and satisfied. While the extra mouthful wouldn't fill you up anyway, you're beginning to challenge your brain to accept that it's OK to stop eating when you're full, even if there is food left over. If you don't feel like eating any more, remind yourself that you don't have to finish everything on your plate if you don't want to.

NEXT TIME YOU ARE HUNGRY, ASK YOURSELF: DO I FEEL? ...

- Emptiness in my stomach
- Dizziness
- Lightheadedness
- A strange feeling in my stomach
- Lack of concentration
- Gurgling, grumbling or rumbling in my stomach
- Tired
- Low in energy
- A headache
- Nausea

What does hungry feel like?

Still not 100 per cent comfortable identifying what hunger feels like for you? Don't worry! Even after years of trying every diet, it can still take time. With practice, you'll get better at reading your appetite, eating when you're hungry and stopping when you feel satisfied.

Hunger feels different for different people. So what does hunger feel like for you?

Some of these symptoms may only come on once you're quite hungry (9+ on the hunger scale) but with practice, you'll start to notice them earlier. There is no need to panic because hunger doesn't sneak up on you (unless you're really busy and distracted). Physical hunger builds slowly, so you'll notice these symptoms as they grow.

KNOW YOUR HUNGER

- Try not to let yourself get too hungry (0–1), as you're more likely to overeat.
- When you eat until you are overfull (9–10), your stomach is stretched and doesn't feel good.
- Practise keeping your hunger between 3 and 7 on the hunger scale.
- Aim to eat when you are at 3 on the hunger scale.
- Practise finishing your meal when you reach 7 on the hunger scale.
- When you are peckish (4), wait until you are hungry to eat.
- Don't eat by the clock. Stop eating because it's 'meal time' and eat when your body is hungry.
- Work out what hunger feels like for you by noting the signs and symptoms.
- Aim to eat to your hunger most of the time, but allow room to be flexible.
- For the next week, track your hunger using the hunger diary on page 28.

become an intuitive eater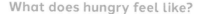

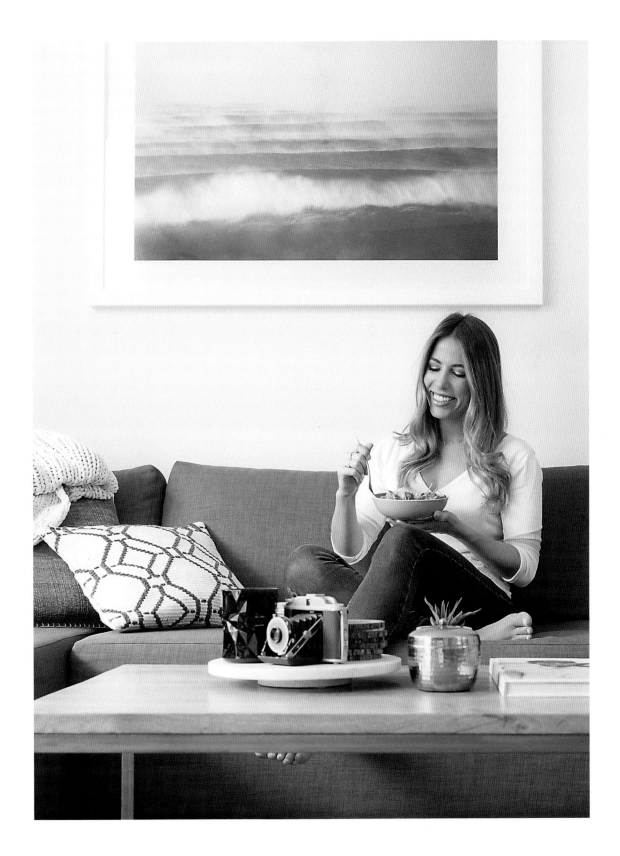

Hunger diary

Photocopy this page and record your hunger for a week.

Before you eat, record your hunger as a number out of 10. Once you've finished eating, write down your hunger rating again. Record what time you eat and what you eat, as well as any exercise you've done. Take note of how long it takes before you become hungry. You may also want to record how you feel, what you are thinking, or any 'wins' you have. For example, you may want to use an asterisk (*) or star to indicate a binge-free meal or day.

   The purpose of keeping a hunger diary is NOT to track how 'good' or 'bad' you are. It's important not to judge what you eat. As you track your hunger, you'll start to see patterns; for example, you may realise you get hungry at around the same time every day or notice that binges happen at a similar time. If recording what you eat feels too restrictive, skip this part. Just try to become more aware of your hunger levels throughout the day.

Use the small boxes to rank your hunger on the hunger scale before each meal: 0 = beyond hungry; 1 = ravenous; 2 = very hungry; 3 = comfortably hungry; 4 = peckish; 5 = neutral; 6 = slightly full; 7 = comfortably full; 8 = quite full; 9= very full; 10 = stuffed, too full.

Date _____   Week number_____

	Monday	Tuesday	Wednesday	Thursday	Friday	Saturday	Sunday
Breakfast Time:							
Snack Time:							
Lunch Time:							
Snack Time:							
Dinner Time:							
Snack Time:							
Exercise							

If you aren't hungry for a meal (even breakfast), you do not need to eat. The healthiest thing to do is to listen to your body and eat when you are hungry.

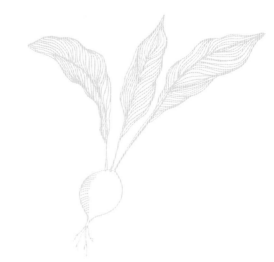

Case study

Michelle

Michelle is a busy mum with three kids under seven. She was constantly dieting but after years of failed diets (which led to secret pantry binges) she decided to tune into her hunger levels instead.

After listening to her hunger for a week, she discovered that she wasn't actually hungry when she woke up at 6:30 am. If she had a morning coffee, she didn't get hungry until around 10 am, well after she got home from dropping the kids at school.

Michelle was confused because she had always been told that breakfast was the most important meal of the day; she made her kids eat breakfast before school for that very reason! When Michelle ate to her hunger and waited until midmorning to have her breakfast, she found she was less hungry throughout the day. She ate lunch later as well, at around 2–3 pm, so she wasn't actually even hungry in the afternoon, which was previously her trickiest time for overeating.

By dinner, she felt comfortably hungry again and could sit down to a meal with her husband. Previously, she would have felt sick from overeating during the afternoon. While Michelle had always been told to eat breakfast first thing to help reduce cravings, she found it made her hungrier. When Michelle started listening to her body instead of the diet rules, she felt good!

Michelle binged less and didn't think about food as much as before. She felt in control and intuitive with food and she didn't spend all day wondering what she was going to eat next. Michelle stopped feeling the need to eat when other people thought it was best for her to eat and instead, ate when her body wanted. Over time, the binge eating stopped. Michelle lost weight, naturally, but the real victory is that she now feels in control and calm around food.

NOT HUNGRY ENOUGH FOR A FULL MEAL? IDEAS FOR HEALTHY SNACKS:

• A handful of nuts
• A banana or an apple (or whatever fruit is in season)
• Coffee
• A green juice
• A glass of milk
• Two boiled eggs

Learning from your hunger diary

Once you've tracked your hunger for a week, use this guide to gather insights and learn about your eating habits.

Step 1. Are you eating when you are hungry?

Use a highlighter or pen to underline any hunger scores lower than two, indicating when you got a little too hungry.

Use a different coloured highlighter or pen to circle hunger scores above three, indicating when you've eaten before you were hungry.

SOLUTIONS: If you're getting too hungry (0–2) more than once a week, try to make your mealtime a little earlier or carry nutritious snacks. Alternatively, you may want to eat a little more at your previous meal. See pages 72–73 to learn how to make a nutritious balanced meal that'll keep you feeling fuller for longer.

If you're eating before you are comfortably hungry (>3), practise waiting an extra half hour. Alternatively, try eating slightly less at your previous meal.

Occasionally you will eat before you're hungry or eat past satiation. Is this happening daily or several times during the week?

Step 2. Look for patterns

You may snack at the same time each day or become overly hungry midmorning, and not yet recognise the pattern. Simply becoming aware of those patterns can help you make a change. See chapter 5 for more tips on managing your eating patterns.

CHALLENGE: You are consistently too hungry (0–1) before eating.
SOLUTIONS: Eat earlier in the day, have a snack between meals or eat a little more at the previous meal.

CHALLENGE: You are consistently not hungry enough (5–10) before a 'meal time'.
SOLUTIONS: Wait a little longer before eating or eat a little less at the previous meal.

CHALLENGE: You eat because you are scared of getting hungry.
SOLUTION: Ask yourself; what is the worst-case scenario? Will I be slightly uncomfortable for a short period? Practise letting yourself experience hunger in a safe environment; for example, on the weekend, when you're at home and don't have other plans.

Step 3. Count your serves of vegies (and fruit)

How many servings of vegetables do you eat per day? Do you manage to get one or two servings of fruit? Could you increase your fresh food intake by even one serve?
SOLUTIONS: Often we fill up on convenience foods instead of reaching for a piece of fruit, such as a banana, even though it's equally convenient. 'Crowding' in more vegetables and fruit is a simple way to feel better. Turn to page 39 for more advice on ways to boost your fresh food intake.

become an intuitive eater

Step 4. Make small tweaks

Now that you're aware of your hunger throughout the day and your eating habits throughout the week, you can start to make small tweaks that can have big effects. As you practise listening to your hunger, you'll get to understand your body more and become more responsive. In the following chapters, I'll be sharing helpful tips to help you to make those powerful yet simple and healthy tweaks.

Ask yourself...

• How long does it take me to move from neutral (5) to comfortably hungry (3) on the hunger scale?

• What times of day am I most in control and comfortable around food?

• What times of day or week am I most vulnerable to overeating?

• Do certain foods keep me feeling fuller for longer?

• Do certain foods make me feel uncomfortable, tired, unwell?

• How many times a day or week am I eating 'sometimes' foods?

• What are three things I can start to do differently?

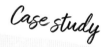

Case study

Valeria

Valeria is a nurse who often works night shifts. At work, she has set meal times. If she is with a patient or in a meeting, she can't start eating an apple, no matter how hungry she is. Valeria was concerned that she wouldn't be able to listen to her hunger. She found she wasn't hungry when she first woke up, but her first work break wasn't until 11 am; by then she was far too hungry and felt dizzy.

Instead of having a full breakfast when she woke up, Valeria decided to listen to her appetite and just have a snack instead. As she wasn't even hungry, Valeria opted for a piece of fruit instead of a bowl of cereal. She found that was all she needed to keep going until her morning break, when she could sit down to eat something more substantial, such as a piece of grainy toast with avocado and a hard-boiled egg. Valeria found that listening to her hunger helped her worry less about food and made her feel good.

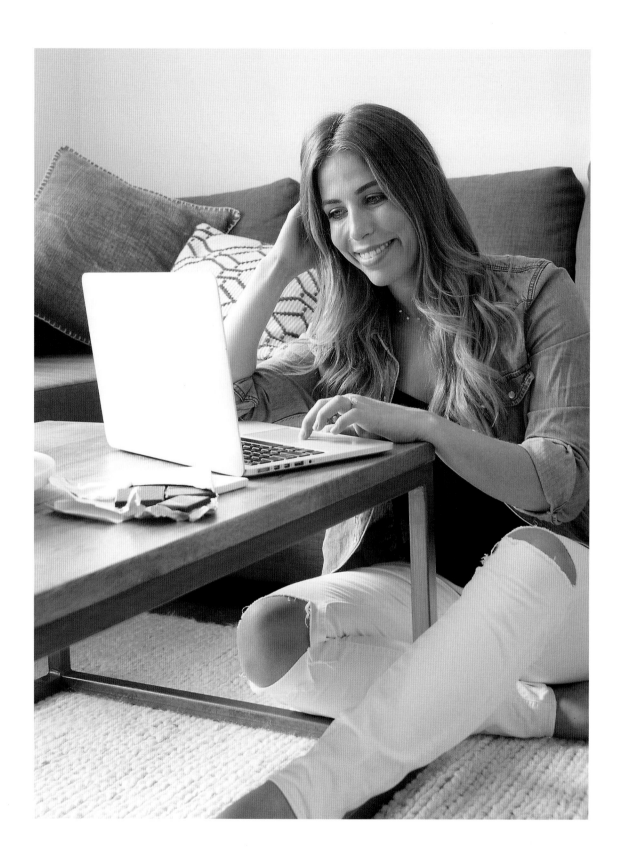

3

Stripped back to *basics*

Nowadays, there is a lot of contradictory advice—and, to be frank, nonsense—that makes it hard to eat well. Luckily, healthy eating is easy when you keep it real, so let's strip the principles of nutrition back to bare basics.

Healthy eating has become complicated, confusing and controversial. But healthy eating doesn't need to be difficult or expensive. Like fashion, the core principles will never change. You certainly don't need to cut out whole food groups, count calories or sell a kidney to pay for overpriced superfoods. Phew!

Health is all about balance. Even if you eat the most nutritious, 'cleanest' diet, if you feel stressed out about food, never feel good about your body or weight and constantly feel deprived, it's not healthy.

THE HEALTHIEST DIET IS FREE FROM:

• Guilt

• Resentment

• Comparison

• Blame

• Deprivation

What is balanced eating?

I aim to eat balanced meals most of the time so that my energy, mood and hormones are more stable and I feel good. Of course, there are dinners out with friends, drinks with colleagues and social arrangements that pop up occasionally, so eating a perfectly balanced diet isn't always going to happen. And that's OK because it's also balanced! I'm not going to miss out on the good things in life just so that I can eat 'perfectly'. Healthy eating is about freedom, flexibility and enjoyment.

I don't like to define how I eat with a label, but I tend to follow a Mediterranean style of eating that includes mostly vegetables,

fruit, wholegrains and legumes, 'healthy' fats from nuts and seeds, avocado and extra virgin olive oil and fish or a bit of meat as a protein source. I'm also a big believer in the adage 'eat everything in moderation'. It's a gloriously simple, flexible and forgiving philosophy that can guide you to eat a balanced diet, although I've got to admit that 'eat everything in moderation' is also a painfully vague expression that can be super impractical, so let's flesh it out!

Eat everything in moderation

What does it even mean? Basically, eat from all the food groups that make YOU feel good.

• Base your diet around vegetables, fruit, wholegrains, seeds and nuts but enjoy a glazed doughnut or a glass of prosecco when it will make you feel good.

• Enjoy the freedom and flexibility to go out with friends and not feel guilty for indulging.

• Never go to extremes. This applies to exercise, supplements, drinking or 'clean eating'.

• Fill up on a variety of foods. Bananas are very good for you, but eating 60 bananas a day doesn't leave room for a variety of nutrients.

• Accept that no single food will break your diet or health. It's the big picture.

The perfect diet doesn't exist. Simply eat food that makes you feel good, energetic and amazing. Sometimes that's a salad. Sometimes that's a piece of cake.

stripped back to basics

TAKE WHAT *works* FOR YOU AND LEAVE THE REST

MY APPROACH:

- Eat real food
- Eat a variety of foods by eating with the seasons
- Eat mostly plants
- Eat food that makes YOU feel good

Find YOUR balance and moderation

Do you feel fine eating foods that contain gluten? Cool. Then don't cut it out. Does lactose agree with you? Great. No need to cut out dairy. Only cut out foods when they don't make you feel good, not because some diet rule tells you that you need to. Instead, throw your hands in the air and yell 'you don't know me' as you take a bite from your home-cooked spaghetti bolognese (see page 166).

Balance is different for everyone and it changes as you change. That's one of the (many) reasons why meal plans don't work. You've got to work out what balance means for you, right now, at this stage in your life.

You'll become your healthiest, most energetic self by responding to your body's needs, not by following the latest trend or celebrity diet. Be picky about what healthy advice you adopt: take what works for you, leave the rest.

Clean eating

The term 'clean eating' has become really popular in recent years. While many 'clean eating' principles, such as eating less processed food and choosing ingredients you recognise, are good advice, 'clean eating' is actually a diet in disguise. Sure, it's not as obvious as other diets, but 'clean eating' comes with a set of rules about what you're allowed to eat. When you eat 'unclean' foods you feel guilty, setting yourself up for an unhealthy relationship with food. It's easy to take 'clean eating' principles to the extreme and many people do, demonising any food that isn't 100 per cent 'clean' and getting stricter and stricter with their rules. It's great to want to eat more nutritious food and fewer processed foods, but there's no need to eat 'clean' when food has never been 'dirty' to start with. Rather, eat food that makes you feel good, fill up on whole foods and enjoy everything in moderation.

Superfoods

The word 'superfood' refers to foods that contain high amounts of nutrients. The term was made up by the media and adopted by the food industry in order to sell more products. It's not a scientific word at all. These days, 'superfoods' are often a weird array of powders, supplements and hard-to-pronounce ingredients; however, the real superfoods are everyday nutritious ingredients, such as fruits, vegetables and legumes, that are found easily

35

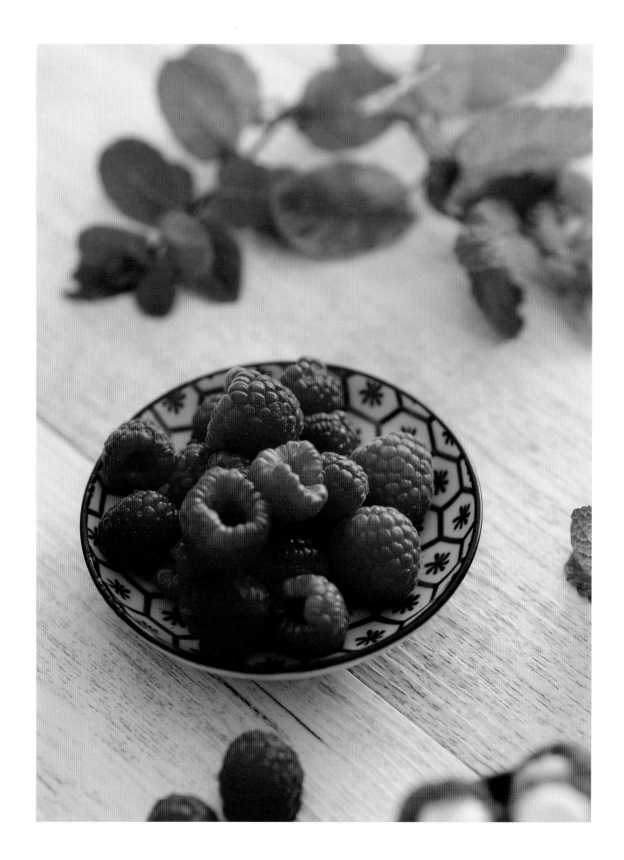

(and cheaply) in your supermarket. Chances are you're completely overestimating how much you need goji berries in your life and completely underestimating the value of vegetables, fruit, nuts and wholegrains. That's the 'superfood' effect!

THE REAL SUPERFOODS ARE:

- **Tomatoes** – loaded with disease-preventing lycopene
- **Spinach and rocket (arugula)** – similar nutritionally to kale, but much easier to eat
- **Berries** – antioxidant powerhouses for reducing inflammation
- **Salmon** – oily fish that fuels the brain with powerful omega-3 fats
- **Nuts (all nuts)** – contain delicious 'healthy' fats that may help balance your hormones
- **Seeds (all seeds)** – plenty of gut-friendly fibre, plus 'healthy' fats
- **Oats** – help lower cholesterol
- **Greek-style yoghurt** – a great source of probiotics

Choosing wholefoods

A wholefood is an ingredient that is as close to its natural state as possible, with minimal processing; for example, a banana is a wholefood, but banana bread is not. Even though a protein powder may contain wholefood ingredients, it is not actually a wholefood. If you can recognise the ingredient without having to read the ingredients list, it's most likely a wholefood. Wholefoods naturally tend to be better for you because they aren't stripped of nutrients (such as fibre, vitamins, minerals and antioxidants) during processing and they don't have additives like sugar, artificial flavours, salt and preservatives.

Unprocessed wholegrains, beans and legumes, milk, fresh fruit and vegetables, nuts and seeds, eggs, fish and meat are all wholefoods. By filling your kitchen with mostly wholefoods, you give yourself a better chance of eating a nutritious meal rather than a fast-food fix.

I try to eat a wholefood-based diet by cooking at home and buying wholefood ingredients. But I live in the real world and not everything I eat can (nor does it have to) be a wholefood. I also eat cheese and yoghurt, bread and breakfast cereals and enjoy sweets and dessert, because I believe in balance.

Vegetables: The main event

I rarely meet anyone who gets their recommended number of vegetable servings daily. According to the latest statistics, only seven per cent of the population eats the recommended five to six serves of vegies a day. Eating more vegetables, not superfoods, might be the single best thing you can do to improve your diet. All other nutrition tips are noise by comparison. Nowadays, I'm a big vegetable lover and I'm always looking for the most vegie-full foods, not the 'cleanest' or lowest in calories. As a result, I naturally end up making healthier choices without the deprivation or restriction. At first, I aimed to eat two to

three serves a day. Then I worked my way up. Some days I don't squeeze five to six serves of vegetables into my diet, but with a bit of hustle, most days I do. And I feel good for it.

WHEN YOU EAT THE RECOMMENDED SERVES OF VEGETABLES:

- Your gut functions better thanks to all the fibre.
- Your immunity is stronger, so you're less likely to get sick.
- Your risk of diseases such as diabetes, heart disease, dementia and even some cancers drops significantly.
- Your energy and mood are boosted.
- Your metabolism speeds up because you're filling up on fibre.
- Your skin looks healthier thanks to antioxidants, nutrients and hydration.
- Your food bill is reduced because you are buying fewer processed foods.
- Your weight is easier to manage.

Load up vegetables

Vegetables should taste freaking delicious. Healthy food needs to feel like a preference, not a chore. Salads and vegetables should never be boring. Because when they are, you end up eating everything except salads, am I right? If adding a drizzle of delicious salad dressing makes you eat more salad, then I am a big fan. I'll be honest: no-one ever got fat from having a drizzle of honey and oil in their salad dressing. It's quite the opposite. Adding salad dressing means you eat more salad and vegetables, helping you maintain a healthy weight. While adding salad dressing (and sauces to vegetables) may add calories, sugar and salt, in the scheme of things, it won't make a material difference.

Did you know salad dressing (apart from tasting yummy) actually boosts the nutritional value of your salad, as the oil helps your body absorb crucial vitamins A, D, E and K from the vegies?

Crazy-delicious salads don't take longer to prepare or require more ingredients than boring old Iceberg lettuce, tomato and cucumber. The art of show-stopping salads is as simple as changing up the combinations. Here some simple four-ingredient salad ideas to take your salads from boring to soaring:

- **Tomato, cucumber, mint, black olives**
- **Rocket (arugula), pear, parmesan, toasted walnuts**
- **Tomato, basil, cucumber, feta cheese**
- **Shredded cabbage, carrot, spring onions (scallions), kale**
- **Chickpeas (garbanzo beans), finely chopped red onion, parsley, tomato**
- **Sweet corn kernels, black beans, tomato, onion**
- **Spinach leaves, strawberries, cucumber, feta cheese**
- **Iceberg lettuce, peas, mint, sunflower seeds**

stripped back to basics

Swap deprivation for crowding

Trying to be 'good' by eating less rubbish doesn't work, because as soon as you cut foods from your diet, you'll feel deprived, start to obsess and crave them even more. When you finally give in to temptation (which is inevitable now that you've turned yourself into a food-crazed lunatic), you'll feel guilty and disappointed. Crowding is much more effective and a positive way to eat healthily. The idea is simple: instead of focusing on the need to cut foods out your diet, simply focus on what you want to add to your diet. Naturally, you'll crowd out the less nutritious options by filling up on the wholesome stuff. It's so simple, it's crazy enough to work. But don't take my word for it. Try it for yourself.

Making even subtle adjustments to how you talk and think about food can make the biggest impact on your eating habits. Here are some crowding mental swaps:

Swap: 'I'm quitting carbohydrates' for 'I'm going to eat an extra serve of vegetables every day'.

Swap: 'I'm not allowed sugar' for 'I'm going to snack on fresh fruit'.

Swap: 'I want to eat less junk' for 'I want to eat food that makes me feel good'.

Swap: 'I can't drink alcohol' for 'I want to wake up with more energy'.

Swap: 'I'm cutting out all processed food' for 'I want to eat more wholefoods'.

Swap: 'I want to eat less fast food' for 'I want to cook more'.

CROWDING BASICS:

- Supercharge with fruit and vegetables. Eat five to 10 serves of vegetables a day. That's a heap of vegetables!
- When you feel like a snack, choose fruit. Eat one or two serves of fruit a day.
- Enjoy a serve of wholegrains with each meal; for example, have oats for breakfast, beans for lunch and brown rice at dinner.
- Eat a serve of legumes every second day or three times a week (if it makes you feel good).
- Have a serve of yoghurt every day (for great probiotics).

Tip

Crowding is a simple way to eat healthily without obsessing or feeling deprived.

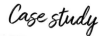

Case study

Andrea

I'm really confused about carbohydrates. Are they fattening? I try to avoid pasta because I've been told it's got too many carbohydrates and isn't healthy. I heard sushi has too much rice and that makes it fattening. Argh! But I love carbs so very much.

It sure is confusing! The health world has hated on carbohydrates for quite a while now, for no good reason. The good news is eating carbohydrates isn't fattening. I'm glad to tell you that pasta and rice are not bad for you. You can certainly eat them as part of your diet. Personally, a life without pasta is not a life I ever intend to live!

Rather than thinking that pasta and sushi have too many carbohydrates, consider the fact that these meals don't provide many vegetables. A salad, for example, will give you up to four serves of veg, but pasta may only provide one serve, on a good day. Sushi may be a great source of 'healthy' fats, and rice is a whole grain but where is the veg? Ordering edamame is great idea, and then you'll maybe reach one serve of veg, but that's about it. Sushi and pasta are healthy options, but eating them every day makes it tricky to get enough variety and vegetables. When ordering pasta or sushi, choose wholemeal versions and find ways to sneak in more vegetables.

Instead of 'what bad things should I avoid?' start to think of 'how can I get more variety or eat more vegetables?' This is a slightly different way of looking at food.

Smuggle in more vegetables

Here are some non-sucky ways to get more veg into your diet.

- Add a handful of spinach leaves to your smoothie (see page 150)
- Put a punnet of sweet baby tomatoes on the kitchen counter for easy snacking.
- Cook up mushrooms, tomatoes, spinach and onion with your eggs.
- Sneak blended zucchini, mushrooms and onion into meatballs or mince.
- Snack on pickles.
- Buy vegetables you actually enjoy eating.
- Base your meal around vegetables or salad (not the meat or carbs).
- Make dip with vegies like spinach, broccoli or tomato.
- Add an extra tin of tomato to casseroles.
- Order edamame with Japanese food.
- Always order a side of vegetables or salad.
- Add corn, baby broccoli (broccolini), eggplant (aubergine) and capsicum (peppers) to the barbecue when you're grilling meat.
- Build delicious salads and use a scrumptious dressing (see page 205).

What about starchy vegetables?

For years I was told that starchy vegetables had too many carbohydrates and were fattening. I believed this dodgy advice and worried that eating vegetables like sweet potato, corn and peas would make me fat. I added these vegetables to the growing list of foods I wasn't allowed to eat and stuck to so-called 'free' vegetables. It wasn't until years later that I realised how unhealthy this advice was.

The first thing I realised was that no-one struggles with their weight because they eat corn on the cob, fresh crispy peas and baked sweet potato. While these vegetables contain carbohydrates, they also contain plenty of fibre (especially loaded in the skin) and antioxidants, a dead giveaway in their bright colour. Vegetables and fruit are an incredibly

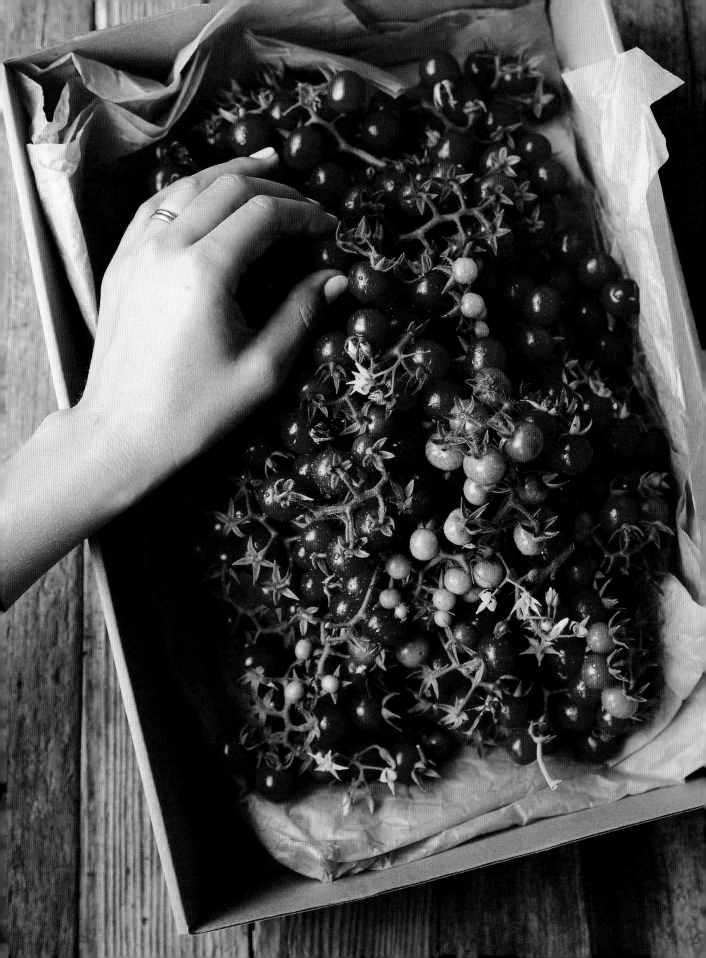

great source of carbohydrates. Arguably, the best there is! Carbs power your body with energy, nutrients and antioxidants and they're cheap and easy to cook.

There are no good or bad vegetables. All vegetables are nutritious and you should eat them all, including the starchier types. The not-so-secret secret is to get plenty of variety.

Eat with the seasons

Seasonal shopping will keep your diet constantly varied so you never fall into a deep, dark food rut. You'll always have new foods to inspire you to eat healthily. Produce grown in the country you live in is almost always going to be in season, cheap or discounted. So you'll save money, support the environment and score the best tasting fruit and veg.

Eat the rainbow

Different coloured fruit and vegetables contain different nutrients. For example, red vegies such as tomatoes contain heart-healthy lycopene, while purple berries are bursting with anthocyanin, a powerful anti-inflammatory. Typically the brighter and deeper the colour, the more antioxidants. For example, baby spinach knocks the socks off iceberg lettuce in the nutrient stakes.

Try something new

We all get into patterns of buying the same old boring fruit and veg at the grocery store. Try buying one new fruit or vegetable each time you shop. Try squash, eggplant (aubergine) or okra. Once home, simply search the web to find a dead-easy recipe and have fun playing.

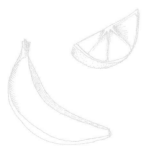

Is it OK to eat frozen or tinned produce?

Yes! Eating frozen and tinned produce can be really convenient and still really good for you! While you might get slightly more nutrients in fresh produce, the nutritional differences are pretty insignificant. The real win is that you snuck in another (convenient) serve of veg. Hooray! You've got to do what's convenient and practical for you in your life, otherwise you'll end up eating cereal for dinner with sad, wilted vegetables at the bottom of your fridge. I like to keep it real—#keepitreal—so I buy a mix of fresh, frozen and tinned produce, which helps me fill up on plenty of fruit and vegetables.

Choosing organic

Eating organic is not worth mortgaging your house for. But if you can afford it, then go for it. Prioritise buying organic fruit and vegetables that you eat with the skin on, such as berries, grapes, zucchini, cucumber, apples and leafy greens and wash it well before eating. Produce such as bananas, avocados and mangoes are less of a priority. When it comes to meat and animal products, I am happy to spend more on hormone-free and organic options. In Australia, for example, most meat is required to be hormone free, but do check the regulations in your country.

I always buy free-range chicken and eggs. Ten thousand hens per hectare is a good guide for free-range, but look for even lower stocking densities if you can.

Fruit is not fattening

I was told that there were good fruits (low in sugar and calories) and bad fruits, so I mistakenly avoided some fruits. But fruit is NOT fattening. Fruit is a wholefood and it's a wonderfully convenient and nutritious snack. Seasonal fruit is affordable and budget friendly. Eating the recommend daily two serves of fruit will help lower your risk of disease thanks to all those lovely antioxidants.

NO-ONE GETS FAT FROM EATING *too much* FRUIT

Most fruits are an incredible source of fibre, helping your gut function at its best and slowing digestion further. Eating fruit (and vegetables) with the skin on is a simple way to get more fibre into your diet and feed the good bacteria in your gut. (Just make sure you wash it well first.) And as fruit comes wrapped in its own skin, it doesn't need a wrapper, so it's also a big win for the environment.

When 50 per cent of the population doesn't eat the recommended amount of fruit each day, the problem is that we are eating less fruit and way more processed high-energy junk food. When you get a sugar craving, fruit is the ideal snack to satiate your taste buds. Make fruit off-limits and you'll end up eating more 'sometimes' food than when you have free reign with fruit. While it's really easy to eat five handfuls of nuts or ten billion bliss balls, eating five apples is more of a challenge. Even though fruit contains sugar, you'd be amazed how much more quickly fruit will fill you up than other snacks. As with vegetables, no-one gets fat from eating too much fruit.

Fruit does contain sugar, but fear not, it's fructose, which is slow burning and reacts differently in your body when packaged in a whole piece of fruit. Some fruits are naturally higher in sugar than others, but all contain this slow-burning sugar that will give you longer-lasting energy than a quick sugar hit from a candy bar. Unlike what the media makes you think, you don't need to buy punnets of blueberries, acai or goji berries to get an antioxidant boost and feel amazing. Eat fruit you enjoy, and that you can afford. Eat fruits with the season and you'll never get bored.

Is dried fruit nutritious?

One of the things that makes fruit filling is that it's made up of loads of water. When you dehydrate or dry out fruit it shrinks, making it less satiating and smaller, so you'll want to eat more to fill up. Fresh fruit is best. But does that mean you should avoid dried fruit? No way. Choose fresh fruit most of the time and when you eat dried fruit, opt for no-added-sugar varieties. Grabbing a family-size bag of dried fruit and snacking on it from your desk is a recipe for overeating. If a handful of dried fruit doesn't satiate you, then next time reach for a whole piece of fresh fruit instead. If you're hungry, then eat substantial, non-snack food, such as a piece of grainy toast with delicious toppings (see page 153).

What about fruit juice?

If you've ever squeezed your own orange juice, you'll know that it takes at least six oranges to make one cup of juice! While it's easy to drink a glass of juice (and not even feel full or satiated), it's much more difficult and would take a lot longer to eat six whole oranges. Juicing also removes the fibre from the fruit. Fibre keeps your gut healthy and requires chewing, helping you to feel full when you're done. Eat whole fruit daily and keep fruit juice as an occasional or 'sometimes' option.

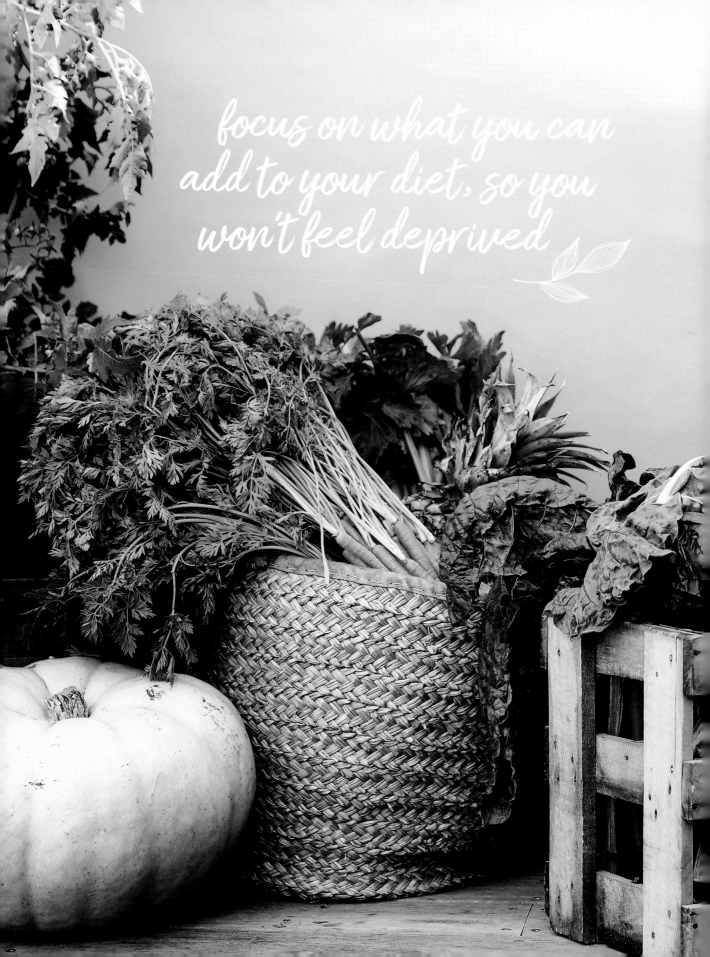

focus on what you can add to your diet, so you won't feel deprived

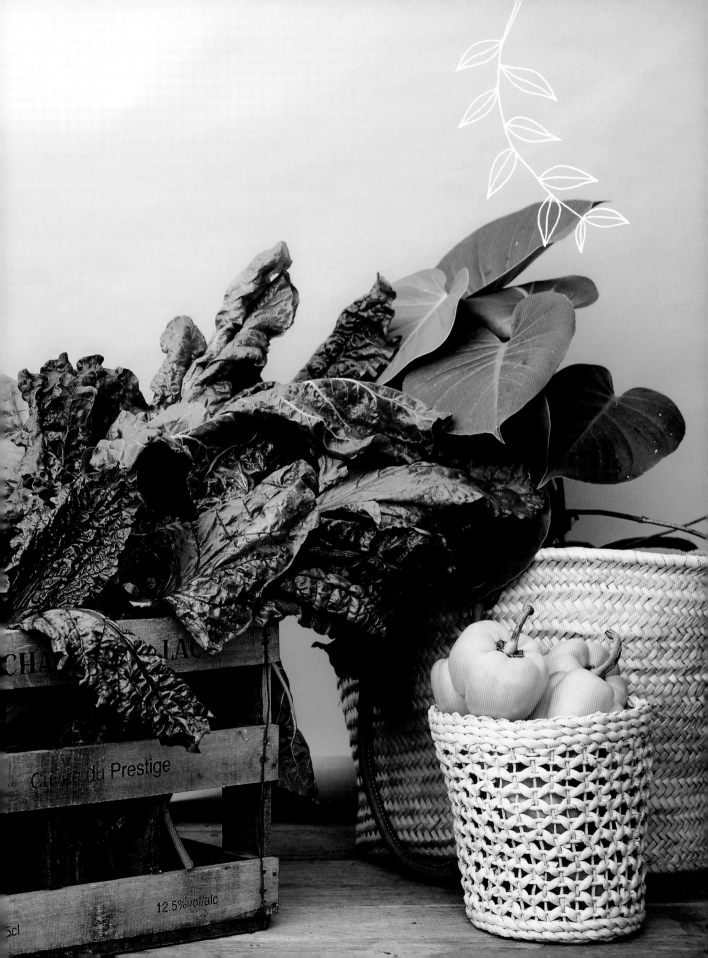

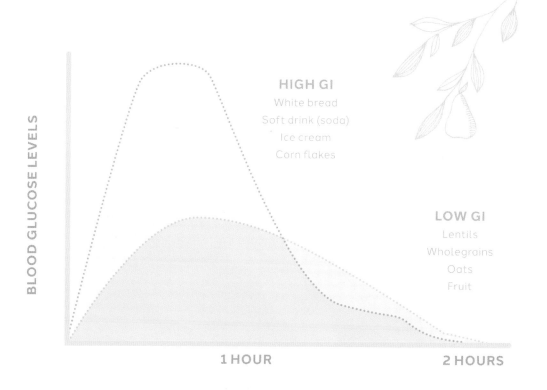

BLOOD GLUCOSE LEVELS

HIGH GI
White bread
Soft drink (soda)
Ice cream
Corn flakes

LOW GI
Lentils
Wholegrains
Oats
Fruit

1 HOUR

2 HOURS

This nifty chart shows how different carbohydrates affect your energy levels. Low GI foods are best to eat every day as they give longer-lasting energy.

CHOOSE SMART CARBS MOST OFTEN. HERE ARE SOME EXAMPLES:

- Wholegrains: oats, freekeh, quinoa, rice, barley, bran
- Fruit (all fruit!)
- Vegetables: especially sweet potato, peas, corn
- Beans and legumes: chickpeas (garbanzo beans), black beans, lentils
- Wholegrain bread
- Dairy: milk, plain yoghurt

Carbohydrates

We've been told to cut out carbs in order to lose weight but it's really not necessary. Yes, you can lose weight from cutting carbohydrates (just like you'll lose weight from cutting out fat, protein or alcohol), but do you want to avoid carbohydrates for the rest of your life? I don't! Carb-phobia won't help you get healthy and stay that way.

Carbohydrates can be nutritious and are a great source of fibre. By choosing healthier, slower-burning and less-processed carbs over refined options, you'll naturally fill up, sideline your cravings and have energy to do the things you love.

The Glycemic Index (GI) is a measure of how quickly foods with carbohydrates are digested and how they affect your blood-sugar levels. The lower the glycemic index of a food, the more steady and longlasting the energy. Smart carbs tend to be low GI, while fast carbs cause big spikes (followed by plummeting lows) in your blood-sugar levels, leaving you feeling moody, tired and irritable. Look for low

stripped back to basics

Casey

When I'm tired or emotional or just plain hungry, I crave carbohydrates. Why is this? I would love to crave a salad, but all I really feel like is a bowl of cereal, a toasted cheese sandwich or two-minute noodles.

That's completely normal. Carbohydrates are your body's preferred energy source because it finds them the easiest to use. When you eat fat or protein, it takes longer for your body to digest and use the energy. Eating carbs also releases serotonin, a hormone that makes you feel better. It's easy to get into a habit of choosing carbohydrates to lift you up, particularly when you're feeling emotional or tired.

Many carbohydrates, such as bread and breakfast cereals, are quick to prepare, cheap and convenient. When you're hungry, every minute seems to matter. So you might also be reaching for carbohydrates because they'll give you fuel faster.

By keeping nutritious, prepped and convenient options in your kitchen, you'll be more likely to reach for vegie-rich meals when you feel this way. If you come home hungry, tired and emotional and open the fridge to find a nutritious, balanced (and delicious) meal ready to eat, the cheese toastie might lose some of its appeal.

Also, remember that carbohydrates aren't bad. Having a hit of unrefined, slow-burning carbs, such as fruit, chickpeas (garbanzo beans), oats, brown rice or a slice of grainy bread, is a great way to balance your meals. And occasionally, you might just make yourself a cheese toastie or pour a bowl of cereal, and that's perfectly fine too.

GI options but keep in mind that low GI doesn't always mean healthy, so consider the overall nutrition of the product.

Slow-burning 'smart' carbohydrates (also referred to as complex or low GI carbs) give you longer-lasting energy, help keep you feeling full, push away cravings, leave you feeling satisfied and prevent energy slumps. Smart carbs tend to be less-refined wholefoods, closer to their natural state.

Fast-burning (or simple) carbohydrates tend to be high GI, meaning your body digests them more quickly, causing a spike in your blood sugar (and insulin) levels. While you'll feel a buzz from the sugar high, the energy will leave you as quickly as it came. Fast carbs deliver a short-term fix and make you feel good whereas smart carbs help you go the distance and keep you feeling good. Many fast carbs are processed and have been stripped of nutrients, such as fibre. Here are some examples:

- **Lollies (candy or sweets)**
- **Soft drinks (soda)**
- **Cakes, cookies and pastries**
- **Refined carbs (white pasta, bread and rice)**
- **Fruit juice and cordial**
- **Sugary breakfast cereals**

Fibre

Adding more fibre to your diet is a dead-easy way to manage your weight without ever feeling deprived. Eating a diet that's high in fibre will help you feel full (thanks to the roughage and bulk) so you end up consuming fewer calories, have comfortable bowel movements and maintain healthy gut bacteria to boost immunity, mood and energy. Fibre is most abundantly found in the skin of fruit and veg (another reason to up your intake) along with legumes and beans, nuts and seeds, popcorn and wholegrains such as quinoa, brown rice and freekeh. Your body does best with 25–30 g (1 oz) of fibre per day. I'm not going to lie, that is a lot of fibre! Processed foods don't contain much fibre, so by simply aiming to eat more fibre in your diet, you'll naturally eat less processed food, cook more at home and load up on plenty more goodness. To increase your fibre intake, choose wholegrain options whenever possible, eat the skin of fruit and vegies and sneak beans, seeds and nuts into meals, such as salads.

Sugar

There is no doubt about it. Eating too much sugar isn't good for your health. A high-sugar diet containing soft drinks (soda), lollies (candy or sweets), processed foods and fast food options accelerates the ageing process, can lead to weight gain, inflammation and diseases as well as unhealthy skin... and it won't make you feel amazing. All sugars cause a spike in your blood-sugar levels. Some are more slowly released, and this is good news for your blood sugar levels. While I don't believe you need to give up sugar completely or eat only low-fructose fruits, I do think it's a smart idea to eat fewer processed sugary foods and cook more at home. A hundred years ago the average person ate one kilogram (2 lb 4 oz) of sugar per year. These days, we eat 60 kilograms (132 lb) of sugar a year. This mostly comes from processed, packaged and takeaway food. When you focus on eating more wholefoods and cooking at home, you don't need to 'quit sugar' because you're crowding it out with fresher, healthier options. Use the recipes in this book (plus you'll find plenty more at lyndicohen.com/recipes) and get creative in the kitchen!

You'll often see 'sugar-free' recipes with rice malt syrup, coconut sugar or maple syrup, but in reality these are all different types of sugar. Use rice malt syrup if you love it, but don't be tricked into thinking it's sugar-free. It's 100 per cent sugar. I still prefer less-processed options such as dates, maple syrup, local honey and fruit to naturally sweeten my food.

HOW TO EAT LESS SUGAR NATURALLY:

- Cook at home more often. Aim for the majority of meals to be home cooked.
- Skip soft drinks (soda), including 'diet' drinks.
- Don't buy sugary sweets for the house. Buy them when you need them, or enjoy them at social occasions.
- Check the ingredients list. Buy foods without added sugar, syrups or juice.
- Snack on fresh fruit when you crave something sweet.
- Make your own sweet treats with natural sweeteners.

MOST OFTEN, THE CRAVING WILL *disappear* WITHIN THE HOUR

Artificial and natural sweeteners

Including sweeteners in your diet, even the ones without calories, won't help you overcome your cravings for sugar. Artificial and natural sweeteners (such as stevia) are found in diet soft drinks, diet chewing gum or in sweeteners for tea and coffee. When you use sweeteners, you body is tricked into thinking you're consuming something sweet, but it never gets the sugar from the food, so instead of satiating your cravings, you build a taste for sweetness and the cravings increase. I now drink my coffee and tea without sweeteners and I stopped drinking diet soft drinks. As a result, I've reduced my desire for sweet things and I don't get the same level of cravings.

The one-hour trick

Cravings can be really intense, but they often don't last very long. If you give them a bit of breathing room, then they typically disappear. The one-hour trick can help you curb cravings and prevent overeating, particularly after dinner (in front of the TV)! It may sound too simple to work, but it really does. When you get a craving, wait an hour; if, after an hour, you still want to eat the sweet, then enjoy the treat (mindfully, not in front of the TV). Most often, the craving will disappear within the hour. This approach works because you still give yourself permission to eat the treat (you aren't restricting). You are simply creating space to see if the craving subsides. The more you practise doing the one-hour trick, the less intense your cravings will become as you retrain your brain.

CRAVINGS CAN BE CAUSED BY:

- **Hormonal changes.** You may crave different foods at different times of the month. I talk about managing your hormones more on pages 118–121.
- **Sleep deprivation.** When you're overtired, your body craves energy from food, but what it really needs is sleep. Tips for getting more shut-eye are on page 136.
- **Habits.** This is the most common cause of cravings. If you get cravings at the same time every day (for example, in the afternoon or after dinner) or when you're in a certain spot (such as while you are driving) then it's most likely that your cravings are formed by habit. Each time you give in to your cravings, you condition your brain to think it will get a hit of energy. Luckily, you can create new habits and break your sugar cravings.

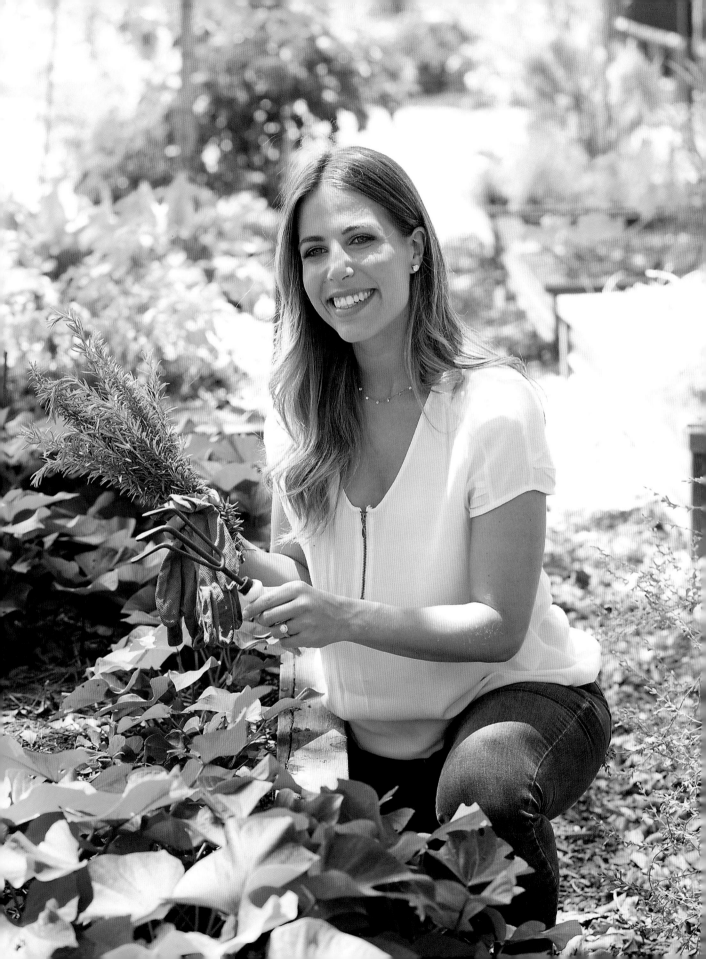

Bliss balls, or protein balls, often provide lots of energy and not much protein. If I make a batch of bliss balls, they are so delicious that I blink and I have devoured the batch... oops! I get around this by freezing them and defrosting them one at a time, buying them individually or making a batch for a friend and keeping just a couple for myself. Alternatively, a piece of fruit is always a healthy snack.

Protein

Protein is broken down into amino acids, which are the building blocks for muscle, hair, fingernails and cells. Protein is a diet essential because it feeds your body, fuels chemical processes and keeps your immune system strong. I'm sure you've heard that eating protein-rich foods such as eggs, nuts and seeds, soy, legumes and beans, dairy and meat helps you feel fuller for longer by slowing digestion and research suggests that protein can help you manage your weight. Eating a variety of foods containing protein by mixing up your diet will help you get all the essential amino acids, including the ones your body can't produce, such as tryptophan (for serotonin and melatonin) and leucine (for brain function).

I think it's good idea to include protein in your meals, but I also think we've become obsessed with protein! To be healthy, it's recommended that you have 0.8–1 g ($^1/_{32}$ oz) of protein for every kilogram (2 lb 4 oz) that you weigh. So if you weigh 80 kg (176 lb), then you need 64–80 g (about 2–2¾ oz) of protein per day. If you're exercising, then up to 1.2 g of protein per day per kilogram is a fair aim, equaling about 94–96 g (3¼ oz) for an 80 kg person in our example. This is surprisingly simple to achieve when you're eating a balanced diet. No supplements needed!

Meal	Food	Protein
Breakfast	Small tub of yoghurt with oats and seeds	15 g (½ oz)
Morning coffee		4 g ($^1/_8$ oz)
Snack	Handful of nuts	10 g ($^3/_8$ oz)
Lunch	Tuna salad with chickpeas and feta cheese	35 g (1¼ oz)
Snack	Fruit	–
Dinner	Chicken stir-fry with brown rice	30 g (1 oz)
Snack	Cut up fruit	–
TOTAL PROTEIN PER DAY		**94 g (3¼ oz)**

While it's a good idea to include protein in many of your meals, do what makes you feel good. For example, sometimes you will have a salad sandwich without any protein or a meat-free meal. This is fine and healthy. Be relaxed with food.

EAT A VARIETY OF FOOD, *mix up* YOUR DIET AND DON'T HAVE TOO MUCH OF ANYTHING

Protein powders

I'm not a fan of protein powders. This is because I prefer to eat real food and protein powders are pretty processed, even the 'better' ones. I also think many people use protein powders when they would do much better snacking on real food, such as protein-rich eggs, nuts and seeds, soy and tofu, beans, dairy foods and occasionally meat.

Dairy foods

I really love the nutritional benefits of dairy. Dairy is such a great source of calcium and protein, plus it tastes great. I drink cow's milk, as I feel good when I have it and my gut doesn't get upset. If you don't feel good on dairy, maybe it's not for you. Speak with your doctor or a dietitian.

Compared with dairy milk, alternatives such as soy or almond milk don't have as much protein or calcium so you'll need to add these essential nutrients into your diet in other ways. Of the alternatives, I believe soy or oat milks are the most nutritious. A glass of soy milk each day is fine for your hormones (see page 121 for more information about hormones), but—as with all things— make sure that you eat a variety of food, mix up your diet and don't have too much of anything.

Full-fat or low-fat dairy: choose the one you enjoy and that makes you feel good. When you cut out fat from a product you lose flavour, so low-fat food will often have added ingredients. Choosing the full-fat version may also help you feel more satiated after eating. Because of this I tend to buy full-fat products, although as I was raised on 'fat-free' options, some full-fat products taste too rich for me.

Rather than only buying one or the other, I eat the one that will make me feel good. Your body's innate ability to help you eat well for your own needs is the best resource to rely on.

Fat

Eating fat does not make you fat. In fact, fat is incredibly important in your diet. Fat fuels your metabolism, helps regulate your hormones and helps you absorb nutrients such as vitamins A, D, E and K. When you eat fat as part of a meal, it helps release hormones that switch off hunger. This may explain why 'French people don't get fat' (they enjoy good amounts of fat in their diet) and why most people in the developed world gain weight despite eating low-fat foods. Cutting out fat from your diet may drive you to eat more of other foods such as carbohydrates, sugars and protein. This creates an imbalance. I don't believe in cutting out anything, including fat. Balance is key.

How much fat should you be eating? We are all different. Some people thrive with more fat while some do better with less. Use your appetite to find what works for you. I like to add a bit of 'healthy' fat to each meal as it's satiating and a great way to fuel my body. Instead of cutting out fat or loading up on low-fat diet food, simply choose better-for-you fats.

There are two different types of fat: unsaturated (including mono- and polyunsaturated) and saturated. Saturated fat, found in many processed foods and especially fried fast food, may increase 'bad' cholesterol levels and can clog arteries. Saturated fat is often hard at room temperature. Unsaturated fats are often liquid

stripped back to basics

at room temperature—for example, extra virgin olive oil—and often come from plants. Unsaturated fats tend to be better for your health and promote 'good' cholesterol levels. Omega–3s are a type of polyunsaturated fat found in high doses in oily fish. Omega–3 fatty acids are fantastic for your health, particularly your brain function (better concentration and memory)! Omega–6s are another type of polyunsaturated fats found mostly in vegetable seed oils. While getting some omega–6s is good for your metabolism, bone and skin health, the healthiest diet will contain more omega–3s than omega–6s. To boost your omega–3 intake, start by cooking more and relying less on fast foods and processed foods. You can also add some great sources of 'healthy' fats to your diet:

- Avocado
- Extra virgin olive oil
- Oily fish such as salmon, trout, sardines (great for omega–3s)
- Nuts and seeds. All nuts and seeds are nutritious so choose a variety!
- Eggs (including the yolk)
- Macadamia and avocado oil

'Healthy' fats provide your body with a fantastic source of energy, help your hair grow shinier, your nails stronger and fuel your hormones.

Cooking oil

I use a high-quality extra virgin olive oil every day in my recipes because it contains the 'healthy' fats that are protective for you, helping you live longer. The words 'extra virgin' basically mean 'top quality'. Unlike regular olive oil, extra virgin olive oil is high in antioxidants, which keeps the oil stable at high temperatures, up to 210°C (410°F), making extra virgin olive oil safe and nutritious for cooking. Store the oil in a dark, cool place (that is, not above your stove) such as a pantry. Buy smaller bottles and use it within six weeks of opening the bottle so you minimise the loss of antioxidants.

WHAT ABOUT COCONUT OIL?

Coconut oil is very popular at the moment, although it's an ingredient I use occasionally, rather than every day. I don't think eating coconut oil will kill you, but I also don't think it's a miracle food that helps you lose weight and live longer (there's yet to be any research that truly backs this up). Use coconut oil if you like, or give it a miss if it's not your jam. Putting coconut oil on your hair and skin can be very nourishing: just be careful not to do it before you go into the sun as you can burn!

Coffee

I believe coffee can be a part of your healthy diet! In fact, thanks to the caffeine in coffee, drinking a cup of joe in the morning can help with memory retention[1] and protect against some diseases including diabetes and liver cancer[2]. I enjoy a cup of coffee in the morning with a bit of milk and no sugar or sweeteners.

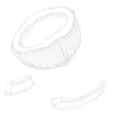

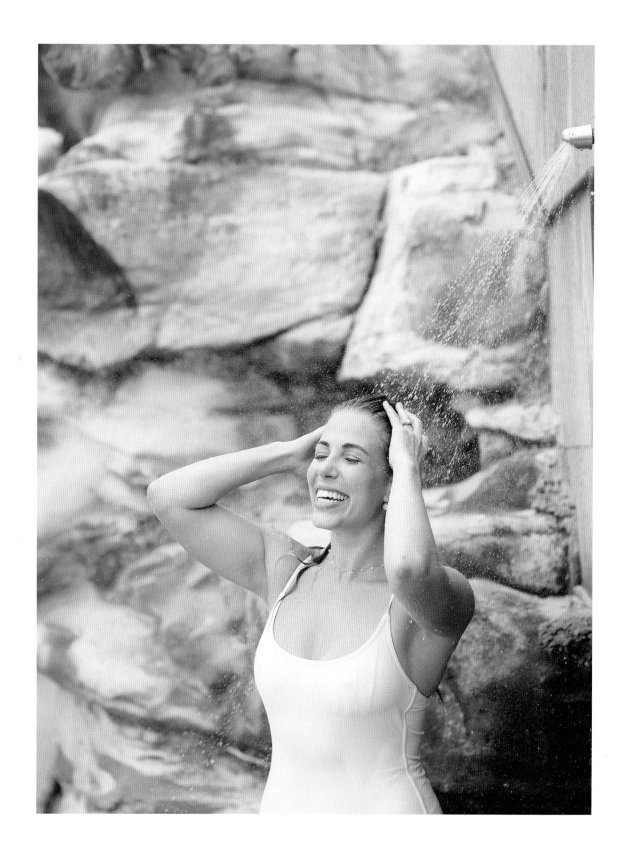

How to *keep it real*

You live in the real world, right? So you need practical tips that really work to get where you want to be, not pseudoscience or unrealistic and outdated health advice. From now on, let's keep it real. Pinky promise, it's real easy—and way more fun. The best bit is that you can go to bed feeling at peace with yourself, and you'll no longer fall off the wagon.

The #keepitreal mindset can help you stay healthy, without dieting or getting obsessed. It's realistic, doable and deliciously enjoyable. In this chapter, I'm going to share with you the key health habits and mindset shifts that will help you keep it real.

I'm assuming that like me, you don't have a maid, a personal chef, an on-hand dietitian or a full-time personal trainer, assistant and stylist waiting on your every need (but wouldn't that be fab?) Our lives are busy and, sometimes, just getting through the day is an accomplishment. Unlike celebrities and Instagram stars, we live in the real world, which means unrealistic health goals and extreme plans don't work because they're simply too difficult, too un-fun and too much freakin' work to keep up with. I'm getting exhausted just thinking about it.

Keeping it real—#keepitreal—is about accepting that you live in the real world. While your health is important, so is your social life and you need to let loose every so often. When you keep it real, you don't sweat the small stuff. When you keep it real, you're happy to take shortcuts to make your life easier, even if it means letting go of perfection, because keeping it real is far better than completely losing your mind and crying yourself to sleep. You understand that small changes really do make a big difference and that if you enjoy the process, you'll never fall off the wagon.

A healthy weight

Weight loss is often pushed at us as the way to get healthier, reduce our risk of diseases such as diabetes and heart disease and live longer, but when I looked a little closer, I was so surprised to learn that there isn't much evidence to back this up. For years, I thought being outside the ideal weight range put you at a much higher risk. But it turns out that there isn't strong evidence that being in the 'normal' weight range is healthier. Can you believe that? What matters more than body weight is having a healthy body, which is much better measured in terms of your cholesterol levels, blood pressure, blood composition and psychological tests than the number on the scale.

Here's the truth. Long-term studies[1,2] find that people with the lowest risk of mortality are in both the 'normal' and 'overweight' body mass index categories. While being either underweight or obese are definitely risk factors for early mortality, being overweight is not associated with a lower life expectancy and in fact the risk is decreasing[3], probably because of better medical care. Focussing on weight loss as the end goal generally makes you less healthy because you're more likely to yo-yo diet, restrict whole food groups, or adopt extreme and unhealthy behaviours to lose weight. This causes inevitable weight regain (plus more). It's no surprise that yo-yo dieting is also associated with depression and having an eating disorder.

OUR CURRENT BEAUTY STANDARD IS *warped*

Get this: research shows that yo-yo dieting is far more unhealthy than maintaining an overweight body mass index (BMI) when it comes to your heart and mental health[4].

We live in a society that shames people who are fat and applauds the skinny, with no value placed on real health. We assume thin is healthy and fat is unhealthy. Our culture shames excess weight so much that at some point, you think to yourself, 'What's the point? I need to lose so much weight and that's too difficult. Why bother?'

If you carry a little more weight than society deems OK, you feel judged and ashamed. Weight stigma keeps you stuck in unhealthy patterns with poor self esteem. Weight stigma prevents you going out with friends, exercising in public or going to the doctor for fear of being shamed. As a result, your health and happiness suffers.

When people diet, they mostly adopt healthier lifestyles, eat nutritious foods such as vegetables and wholegrains and move more, which leads to lower cholesterol, better blood-sugar levels and so on. But because of weight stigma and thin bias, weightloss is always hailed as the important result, rather than the healthy behaviour changes.

What if your weight isn't the problem at all? What if you stopped constantly trying to lose weight and focussed your energy on adopting healthy habits instead? First up, let me challenge your understanding of what a healthy body looks like.

What healthy looks like

It's easy to think that someone with the 'perfect' looking body (by our social standards) is automatically healthy, but that would be a big mistake. For most people born without the model gene (not a real gene, but you get the point!), maintaining the ideal body type often requires extremely unhealthy behaviour. Actor Hugh Jackman has shared in interviews that getting ready for his roles as Wolverine involved intense training regimes, strict eating and severe dehydration to get the ripped, lean and so-called 'healthy' look. Men around the globe are desperate to get the same chiselled body, not realising that chasing that 'perfect' body has the potential to cause dizziness, fainting, seizures, kidney damage and death.

For women, it's the same story. Models prepare for prestigious runway shows by undergoing months of rigorous preparation. Foods, including many vegetables, fruits and dairy, are removed from their diets. Days before the show, the models cut out even more food groups and often drink laxative teas. This intense regime is super strict and incredibly unhealthy, yet models are applauded as the picture of beauty and health. What you don't see is the explosive diarrhoea, abdominal cramping and hunger pangs. Not quite as sexy, when you think about it like that!

Our current beauty standard is warped. What we think of as a healthy body can often require very unhealthy strategies to achieve. If you lined up a row of people who actually lived a truly healthy balanced life, you wouldn't see a row of people with the same ultraslim physique. You'd see people of all shapes, including those with soft tummies, cellulite and stretch marks. Most people don't naturally have a bikini body or abs when they are at their healthiest weight. If you've ever watched the Olympics, it's clear that the best athletes in the world come in all shapes and sizes. We need to redefine what a healthy body actually looks like.

Health is not a size. Health is having enough energy to do the things you love. Health is fuelling up with nutritious foods that make you feel good, moving your body and being strong. Health is also about having the flexibility to catch up with friends (even if that means missing a workout) and feeling relaxed around food.

It's normal, in our weight-obsessed culture, to feel the need to have the 'perfect' body. I have bad body-image days as well. I'm not sure you can live in our society, use social media and absorb pop culture and not feel the pressure to be slim. It's intense. But you can also decide that you don't want to be a victim of it, that you want more for yourself and your children. You can decide that you don't believe in the story that you need a low body-fat percentage to be healthy. You can choose to stop chasing an ideal that you cannot maintain, let alone reach. You can decide that you're no longer willing to sacrifice your mental health to lose weight. Don't give up 95 per cent of your life to weigh five per cent less.

My big weight loss secret

I'm always asked, 'how did you lose 20 kg (44 lb) and keep it off? The big secret to my weight loss is that I didn't try to lose weight. It turns out that trying to lose weight was having the opposite effect. Up until my 'Aha' (I-need-to-stop-dieting) moment, I was obsessed with losing weight. It was the only reason I ate salads and exercised. But I finally realised it wasn't working.

Trying to lose weight had made me hate my body and gain weight. So I wondered, what if I stopped trying to lose weight and focussed on being healthy? I calculated the risk. The worst-case scenario was that I would gain more weight and I was so scared—actually terrified—of that happening; but I also realised I needed to make a change. I didn't want to diet for the rest of my life. If dieting had made me gain weight, then maybe not-dieting would do the opposite. What did I have to lose?

So when I say I gave up dieting, I also mean to say that I gave up trying to lose weight. It took an extraordinary effort to resist the temptation to diet. But I trusted myself, practised the principles in this book and started to think about food differently. By about four years later, I had lost 20 kg (44 lb). This weight loss was so slow that I couldn't have measured it with a scale. Averaged out over the period, I lost 100 g (3½ oz) a week. If my goal had been to lose weight, I would have been incredibly disheartened and lost motivation when I stepped on the scale each week. I wouldn't have noticed all the other incredible progress I had made because I would have defined my success by the scale. Without any weight loss, I would have given up.

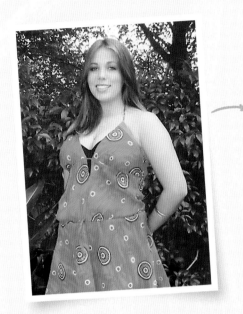

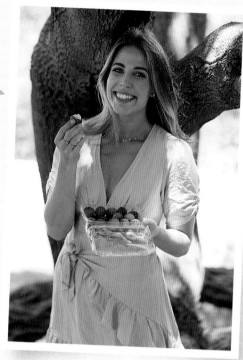

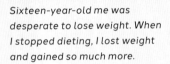
Sixteen-year-old me was desperate to lose weight. When I stopped dieting, I lost weight and gained so much more.

Luckily, I didn't measure my success with a scale. I measured the changes in my relationship with food and my habits. Instead of starting one hundred new habits on the first of January, I adopted habits slowly, one by one, giving my brain, preferences and lifestyle time to change with me. So, while the scale didn't always reflect the healthy changes I was making, my mind slowly changed for the better and, sure enough, my body slowly started to change with it.

Ironically, as long as you define your success by your weight, you won't ever get to your healthiest and be able to stay there. Why? Because when you lose the weight, you feel like you've reached your goal: you get complacent about eating healthily and exercising, as it feels like the battle has been won. When you define success by the number on the scale or the amount you lose in a week, you're setting yourself up for an 'all-or-nothing' approach and, like the majority of people, you will probably fail.

I appreciate that you might not feel that you are currently at your healthiest weight. You find yourself tired, sweaty and uncomfortable in your clothes; you're desperate to shift some weight so you can feel good again. You eat past the point of fullness. But at some point, you need to take a long-term view.

Going on a weight-loss diet is a short-term goal. It's like trying to swim to the other side of a river with a very strong current. You'll get exhausted and the current will end up pulling you back to where you started. On each attempt, you grow weaker and are less successful. Focussing on healthy habits instead is like building a bridge across the river. Yes, it's going to take much longer, but once you've built a solid foundation, getting to the other side is easy and effortless.

Stop wasting energy on short-term weight loss. Aim for long-term health. Stop 'trying to be good' and start trying to feel good.

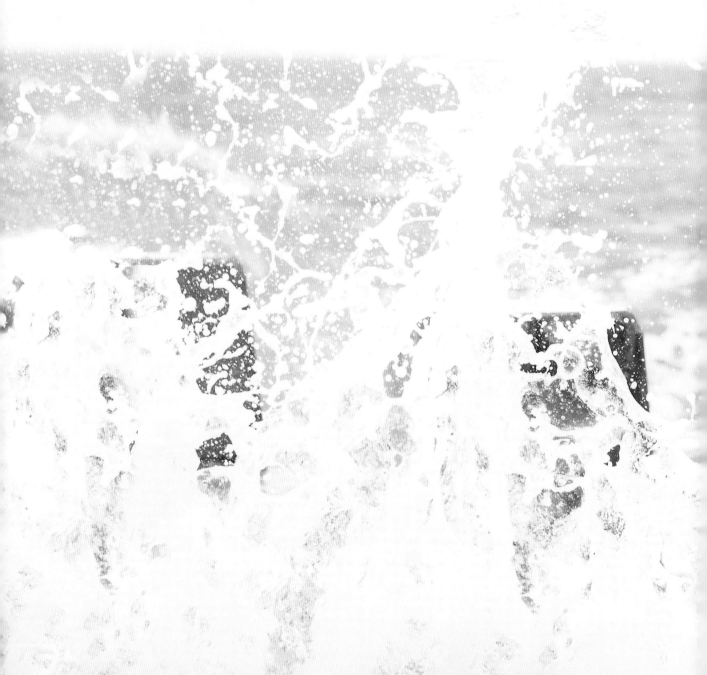

stop 'trying to be good' and start trying to feel good

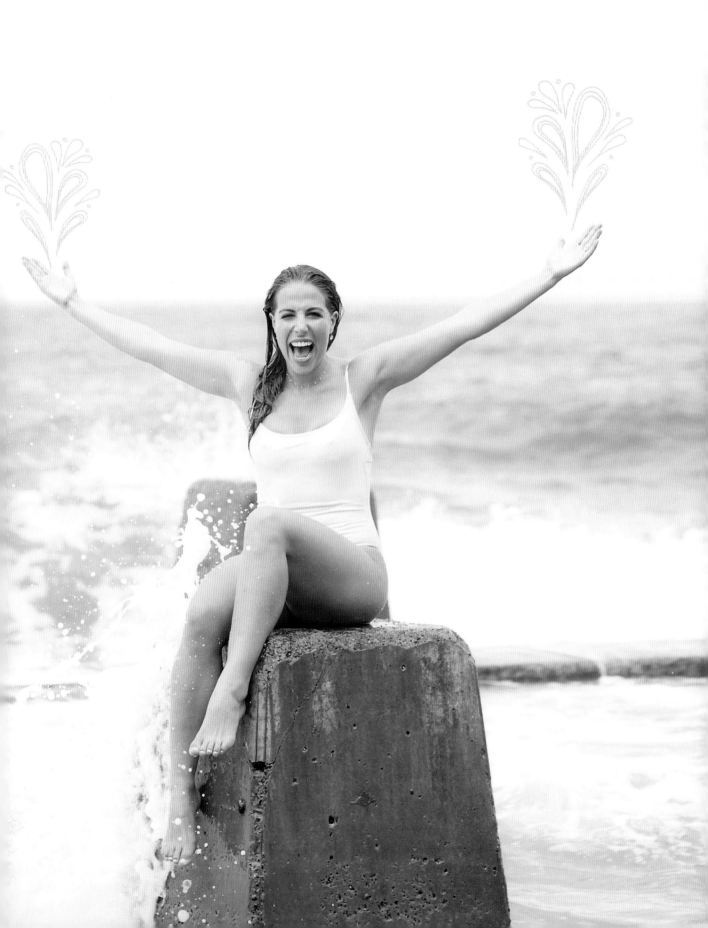

Awesome, non-sucky, life-changing healthy habits you might want to sink your teeth into

1. Add a serve of vegetables to your breakfasts.
2. Aim to take 10,000 steps each day. Download an app or get a fitness tracker to help (but turn off the calorie counter).
3. Cook at home one more night each week.
4. Practise crowding in more healthy food.
5. When you cook dinner, make twice as much, so you can have a healthy lunch the following day.
6. Buy a large water bottle and keep it on your desk or in your bag.
7. When eating a meal, start eating the vegetables first.
8. Halve the amount of sugar in your coffee or tea, or cut back to none.
9. Swap soft drinks (soda) for tea or water.
10. Aim to eat two pieces of fruit every day.
11. Eat when you are hungry, not by the clock.
12. Always take the stairs. Walk when on escalators.
13. Start some enjoyable exercise, whether it's walking, yoga, dancing, weightlifting or a team sport.
14. Embrace a meat-free meal once a week (try 'meat-free Monday').
15. Reduce aimless social media or email checking by deleting apps from your phone.
16. Stop weighing yourself.
17. Make an appointment with a counsellor or psychologist.
18. Swap catching up with friends over coffee or cocktails for catching up on a walk.
19. Fill your shopping trolley with 50 per cent veg and fruit (this way you will eat 50 per cent veg and fruit!)
20. Stop eating in front of the TV.
21. Buy one new healthy ingredient each week that is outside your comfort zone.
22. Go to sleep 30 minutes earlier.
23. Always order a side salad and veg when eating out.
24. Find reasons to walk. Walk to buy your groceries, get off the bus a few stops earlier, or walk for 20 minutes on your lunch break.
25. Start a herb or vegie garden and be inspired to cook more.
26. Unsubscribe from social media accounts or websites that make you feel bad about yourself.
27. Prioritise yourself. Practise saying no so you have more space for you.
28. Eat seasonally by buying 'local' and looking for cheap produce.
29. Eat one cup of legumes each week. Add a tin of chickpeas (garbanzo beans), lentils or black beans to a salad or soup.
30. Embrace 'white space': Try not to check your smart device every few minutes.
31. Order your favourite foods with friends and family rather than eating 'forbidden foods' in private.
32. Invest in a standing desk or set a reminder on your computer to stand up and walk around every couple of hours.
33. Do a healthy grocery shop once or twice a week, or get nutritious groceries delivered.
34. Add one more serve of greens to your dinner plate.
35. Decide to be kinder to yourself. Forgive yourself faster. Judge less.

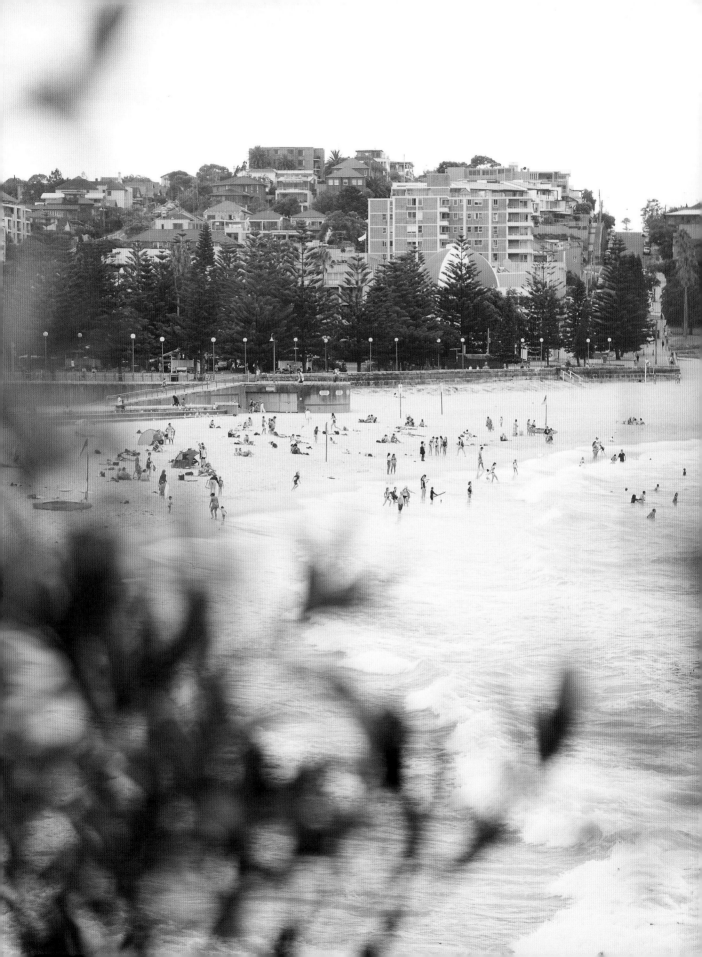

Finding your healthiest weight

Your healthiest weight is not a body mass index (BMI) number, it is the weight you are when you feel strong and have energy to do the things you love. It's the weight you're at when your mood and hormones are balanced and you can do all the things you want to do. Maintaining your healthiest weight never feels like a struggle. It's the weight at which your body feels most comfortable.

Do you know why it's difficult to lose the last few kilograms or pounds? It's because you're probably not supposed to. Those extra kilograms or pounds, that weight where your body naturally wants to be, that's where your body functions at its best. Your hormones are balanced, your body is strong and your mood is stable. It's the weight where you fall asleep easily, have boundless energy during the day and your mind is free to think about things other than macronutrients, calories or reps at the gym.

If it feels like your body is fighting against you when you try to lose that last kilogram, it's because it probably is. When your weight drops, your body will fight back with a slowed metabolism, obsessive thoughts about food and emotional overeating. When you push your body to lose those last few stubborn pounds, you're giving up more than just calories. You miss out on life. You miss out on sharing laughs with your friends over a cheese board or falling asleep easily, feeling satiated. You pay with your freedom, your spontaneity and the simple pleasures in life. You miss out on unforgettable moments and favourite holiday memories.

Stop weighing yourself

Think of all those mornings you've woken up, excited to weigh yourself only to be left disappointed at seeing the 'wrong' number. Think of the destruction the scale has caused to your mood and motivation. Every morning I used to wake up, hop on the scale and allow the number on the scale to dictate my mood and my self-worth for the day. That number defined me! Weighing yourself is not motivating and it doesn't help you lose weight. It sabotages your relationship with food, which causes deeper, psychological weight problems. When you stop weighing yourself, you are liberated from the obsession with numbers. You are more resilient when you make little slip-ups along the way (which are an inevitable part of life), because you are not defined by the number on a scale.

Weigh-ins promote unhealthy behaviours (like smoking, drug use, skipping meals, calorie counting) to lose weight instead of healthy behaviours (such as lifting weights, eating healthy foods and listening to your body).

Take action: It's time to stop weighing yourself. Also, stop letting someone else weigh you for 'check ins' at support groups or your nutritionist's rooms. Give your scale away. Put it in the garage. Or at the very least, put it at the top of a cupboard where it won't tempt you. When your body changes, you will feel it. You may even see it after a while. Trust me, you'll know because you'll feel better. By listening to your body, not measuring with a scale, you can start to rebuild your relationship with food.

HEALTHY HABITS

Adopting healthy habits—the kind that feel easy, doable and fun—is the surest way to your healthiest self. Unlike diets, adopting healthy habits won't make you feel deprived or restricted. In fact, they kinda tend to make you feel freaking amazing.

There is a strategy to keep in mind. You can't go gung-ho and adopt a whole basket of new healthy habits in one fell swoop and expect them all to stick. You'll burn out, get injured, run out of steam, or find it all too complicated. Too much, too soon, not gonna happen. Let's #keepitreal instead.

The trick is to adopt habits one by one and slowly, giving your brain, preferences and lifestyle a chance to keep up. Once you've found a habit that sticks, that feels good, that is easy to do, that has become intuitive, you're ready to adopt the next healthy habit. As you feel ready, you can keep on collecting these habits. Over time, these small healthy habits start to add up, and the results are incredible. One day you look around and you're the person you always wanted to be, no more wishing and hoping. Small changes add up to make a really big difference over time.

While I know you'd love to go from feeling blah to amazing overnight, think of it like learning a new language. You can't expect to speak fluent Spanish after a few weeks or months. You learn a new language word by word. The more you practise, the more intuitive it becomes.

It's the same thing for eating. After years of dieting, it can seem as if you're learning a completely new food language. If you've been dieting for years, it's going to take time and require patience.

Considering quitting sugar or cutting out carbs? First ask yourself: Am I willing to do this for the rest of my life?

If the answer is no, it doesn't how much better you'll feel when doing it: if you can't maintain it for the rest of your life, the results will be short-lived. For example, fasting diets work. But if you don't want to fast every few days for the rest of your life, then don't waste time doing it in the short term. As soon as you stop fasting, you'll regain the weight you lost. If a habit becomes a pain, too hard or makes you feel anything other than amazing, let it go. No shame or guilt. Lesson learned: knowledge gained. There are plenty more healthy habits in the sea. Time to pick another!

Creating a healthy environment

I believe a healthy diet starts with a healthy kitchen. Your environment can either support or hinder you. When your kitchen, pantry and fridge are filled with nutritious options, you

Tip

Don't go shopping hungry as you will buy everything in aisle four. If you need to, have a snack before you go into the shops. A piece of fruit, a handful of nuts or even a sushi roll or sashimi are great choices that can be bought right outside the store. Very hungry? Grab a sandwich from the food court.

won't need to rely on willpower and you'll find it much easier to fill up on salads, vegies, fruit and wholegrains.

Grocery shopping

Nail a healthy grocery shop and you'll find it so much easier to eat healthy during the week. Here is where you can practise 'crowding'. Fill your shopping trolley with mostly vibrant, healthy foods and you'll fill up on those foods.

Use your shopping trolley as a guide. Before checking out, ask yourself: Does the food in my trolley reflect the way I'd like to eat?

I like to fill my trolley with 'everyday' food. If I feel like a treat at home, I'll make something quickly using wholefood ingredients (such as dates, bananas and nuts) and the recipes in this book. I prefer not to buy treats for my house (because I will eat them!) and instead I order dessert or other 'sometimes' foods when eating out or on special occasions.

Walk around the outer aisles of the supermarket as this is where the wholefoods are stored. If there are more items on your list, shop for them with purpose rather than perusing the aisles aimlessly.

MAKE THE MOST OF YOUR FREEZER!

I like to freeze food in portion-sized containers so I don't need to defrost the whole thing. For example, I'll make my Chocolate banana bread (see page 220) and freeze individual slices, ready for a snack. Here are some things you'll find in my freezer:

Frozen seasonal fruit: When fruit is in season, I buy lots at bargain prices and freeze in portion-sized containers ready for a smoothie or healthy sorbet. See recipes on page 223.

Frozen banana, chopped

Frozen grapes (great snack)

Frozen berries

Frozen lime juice: limes can be expensive so buy them up when they are in season and freeze the juice in your icetray.

Edamame beans, shelled (find them in Asian supermarkets)

Cooked meals (from when I have leftovers)

Frozen milk: frozen in icetrays, it's great for thickening a smoothie or when you run out of milk and can't get to the shop.

Frozen herbs: Freeze extra herbs in water, stock or extra virgin olive oil in an icetray.

Start a small herb garden

I live in a small apartment, but I've installed a small herb garden on the wall to grow herbs on my balcony. I also have little pots of herbs around my kitchen, which look so pretty. Mint, spring onions (scallions), basil, parsley, rosemary, thyme and chillies are so easy to grow. Coriander (cilantro) can be a bit tricky! Growing my own herbs saves me so much money. Start by growing your favourite herb in a pot and then grow (literally) from there.

Batch cooking and meal prepping

Investing time to do basic meal prep can make a massive difference to how healthily you eat throughout the week. When your house is filled with ready-to-cook options, you'll eat them.

When it comes to meal prep and batch cooking, you either love it or you want to love it, but you never find time to do it. It can often feel overwhelming and it can be added to the growing list of things you don't have time for.

How about this? If meal prep doesn't suit you, forget it. Don't keep hacking at any health habit and wasting precious headspace on something that doesn't work for you right now. The healthiest way of eating is doing what is easy and enjoyable.

I personally don't do meal prep. Instead I tend to batch cook and choose simple recipes; for example, I make soup on Monday night for dinner and make sure there are plenty of leftovers for the week ahead. But if you love meal prep, here are some ideas:

- Cook whole grains. Alternate each week: my favourites are brown rice, quinoa, freekeh or pots of overnight oats.
- Seasonal soup. Make two or three times the quantity you need for one meal and freeze whatever you won't eat now in portion-sized containers. (See page 174 for a recipe.)
- Slow-cooked meals. I use my slow cooker for delicious curries, stews and other meals.
- Roasted vegetables: perfect for serving with cooked meats, layering on wholegrains

YOU CAN'T ALWAYS COOK EVERYTHING *from scratch*, AND YOU SHOULDN'T FEEL GUILTY WHEN YOU DON'T

or serving on a bed of leafy greens to make an instant salad. Check page 200 for my Lifesaving baked rainbow vegies recipe.

- Toast nuts and seeds in bulk and keep them in an airtight container.
- Chop vegetables, such as carrots, so they are ready to be eaten. Store in airtight containers in the fridge.
- Boil eggs. Add them to salads or sandwiches for lunch. They will last in the fridge for three to four days when kept in their shells.
- Make my Get-up-and-go overnight oats (see page 155) for a week of convenient healthy breakfasts.

Embrace convenient health foods

To help me eat healthily, I rely on some fantastic convenience health foods. These options are great for busy weeks or to simply make healthy eating easier all the time. You can't always cook everything from scratch, and you shouldn't feel guilty when you don't. In fact, you may notice you cook more when you use some convenience options because cooking is faster, easier and more enjoyable.

- Precooked brown rice or quinoa. Easy to warm up in microwavable bags. Keep one or two at work.
- Precut vegetables. If you are really time poor, buy precut vegetables such as pumpkin (squash), onions, zucchini (courgette) noodles, carrot noodles and so on. This can save a lot of time.
- Fresh soup from the cold section of the supermarket. Skip powdered or tinned soup. Buy fresh options and check the ingredients list so you know what's in it.

- Premarinated protein. Scan the ingredients list to see what has been used. If the protein is already marinated, it's easy to cook and pull together a salad.
- Prewashed lettuce leaves. Ready to throw into a salad.
- Roasted free-range chicken. While I'd prefer to cook my own from scratch, these chooks are incredibly convenient.
- Tinned tuna is convenient and tasty. I buy tuna in oil because I prefer the flavour compared with spring water. I drain the oil and then use it as a dressing or to cook with.
- Tinned legumes like chickpeas (garbanzo beans), lentils, four-bean mix. I always have tinned (and dried) legumes on hand to add to soups, salads, dips, stew or to snack on. Rinse drained beans twice to reduce the sodium levels.

Tip

When it comes to your health, find what works for you and ditch the rest. The ability to ignore well-intentioned (but not right for you) advice is potentially the healthiest habit of all.

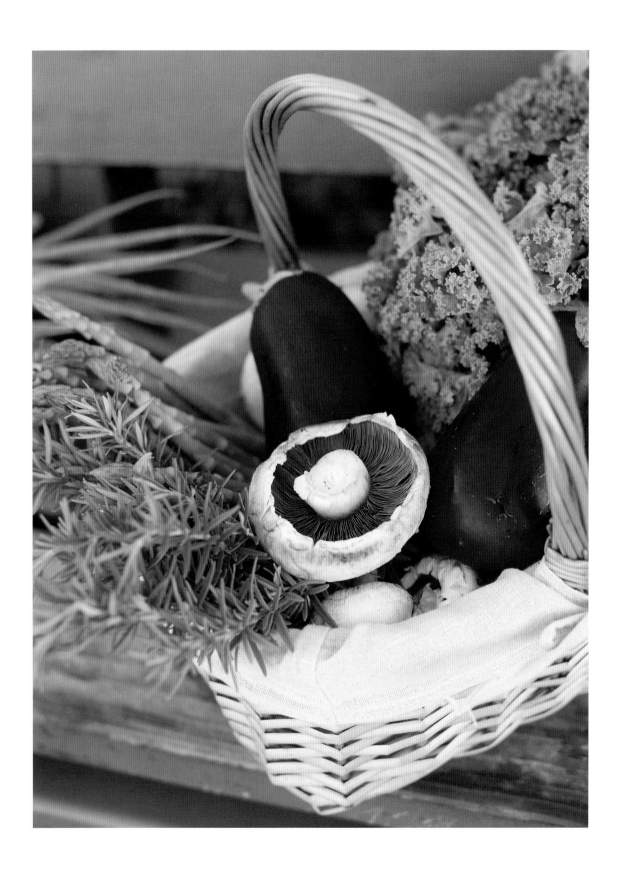

Snacks

I often see recommendations to snack frequently to prevent hunger. For years we were told to have six small meals a day to keep our metabolisms going, but I don't think frequent snacking is a good recommendation for everyone. It's really tough to stop eating once you've started, thanks to the hunger hormones ghrelin and leptin. Some people function best by eating main meals, with maybe one snack (or none) between. At mealtimes they are hungry and finish feeling satiated. Other people need frequent snacks as their blood-sugar levels drop too low between meals. Which style best suits you?

It's a good idea to include a snack, especially in the afternoon, if:

- You get hungry, lightheaded or shaky between meals when you don't eat.
- You get moody in the afternoon or evening. This might be because of low blood-sugar levels.
- You're managing your blood-sugar levels for diabetes. As you have learned, if you are hungry, you should eat – and eat to satiate your hunger.

Many people get into the habit of snacking or grazing, without waiting to feel hungry. Can you relate to these scenarios?

- You snack because it's break time or you 'feel like something'. Snacking has become a habit, rather than a response to hunger. This happens most often in the afternoon, when you start to feel tired or you've had a hard day and feel the need to 'treat yourself' with food. If this is you, then practise waiting until you get hungry to eat. Make a change to your usual routine; for example, go to the gym after work instead of before work.
- You arrive home after work ravenous. Having a satiating snack, such as a quarter of an avocado on toast, before you leave the office can prevent evening binges.
- You don't have a large enough snack. A common mistake is having too small a snack

HEALTHY SNACK IDEAS, DEPENDING ON YOUR HUNGER LEVEL.

Something light

Serve of seasonal fruit such as strawberries, a cup of cherries, a mango, a banana, a pear or two apricots, a bunch of grapes or a large juicy peach

A handful of toasted nuts and seeds

Chopped vegetables with a dip, such as hummus

Small cheese portion

A tub of Greek-style yoghurt

Steamed edamame

An energy ball (bliss ball)

Frozen grapes

A couple of dates with peanut butter and a sprinkle of salt

Toasted chickpeas (garbanzo beans)

More substantial snacks

A piece of grainy toast with a quarter of an avocado, or ricotta and honey, or a tin of tuna

A tub of yoghurt with a handful of seeds, nuts and fresh berries

A small cheese portion on a piece of grainy toast

A bowl of vegetable soup

A brown-rice sushi roll

Salad

A protein bar (see recipe on page 162)

100 g (3½ oz) of ricotta cheese with honey

Chia pudding (see recipe on page 149)

Overnight oats (see recipe on page 155)

Smoothie (see recipe on page 150)

when you are hungry, so you remain hungry. You don't give yourself permission to eat something filling because you're trying to be 'good', then just keep on grazing. Choose a more filling snack, such as a tub of Greek-style yoghurt with a handful of nuts, instead of just having a handful of nuts.

• You aren't hungry for your next meal. If you often find you're not hungry enough for the next meal, you might be snacking because you think you should. Try waiting for your hunger and or make your previous meal or snack slightly lighter.

Portion sizes

Becoming mindful of your portion sizes can help you fuel your body with the energy it needs. You don't need to weigh food, use measuring cups or count calories (I certainly don't). Simply use your hands as an easy way to make mindful portion size choices.

Carbohydrates = size of your clenched fist
Protein = size of your palm, no fingers
Vegetables = size of your clenched fist
Fresh fruit = size of your clenched fist
Oil or fat = size of your thumb
Cheese = size of two thumbs
Nuts = one handful
Avocado = a quarter of a medium avocado

You don't need to learn the exact portion sizes for every food when you use your hand measurements as a rough guide, along with your hunger. Food labels can also sometimes hint to the portion size of the food.

Case study

Anna

This may seem really small, but for as long as I can remember I've never thought one slice of toast would fill me up for breakfast. Even if I had eggs I'd have it with two slices of bread and eat it all up; however, since learning about intuitive eating, I woke up the other day and thought actually all I feel like is one slice of wholegrain toast with some peanut butter. I ate it and was satisfied. I wasn't hungry anymore and it kept me going. One small step for me... #keepitreal

How many serves do I need to have per meal or per day?

How much you need to eat depends on many things like your hunger, hormones, how tall you are and your activity level. Some days you'll need two portions at snack time. Other days, one piece of fruit will satisfy you just fine. And then there will be days when you're not even hungry and you don't need a snack at all. Using my balanced meal guide on the following pages will help you create satiating and balanced meals.

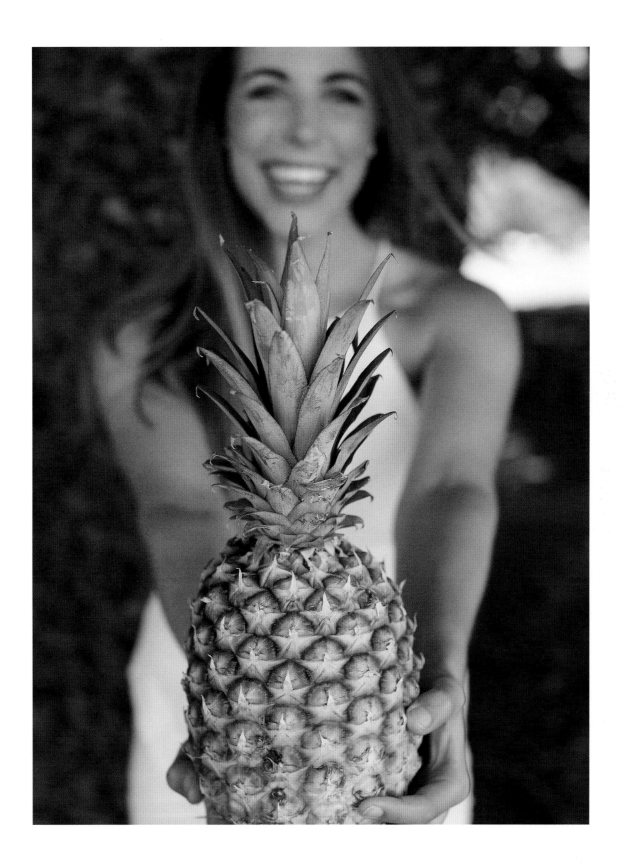

My balanced meal guide

When you're creating balanced meals, you're more likely to feel full and satiated. You'll also get a good mix of nutrients! This simple formula can help you create healthy balanced meals, no matter what you're making. You may notice that when you apply this formula, your meals will keep you feeling fuller for longer, balance your energy, mood and hormones, boost your metabolism and help you feel good.

There are no rules here – this is simply a guide. You won't apply this formula for all meals. Sometimes you might have a bit more protein or fat without the carbs. Other times you may eat only carbohydrates and vegies... and that's OK. Flexibility is important. Let the balanced meal formula guide you, if you find it helpful. If it feels restrictive in any way, ditch it! Simply practise 'crowding' instead (see page 39).

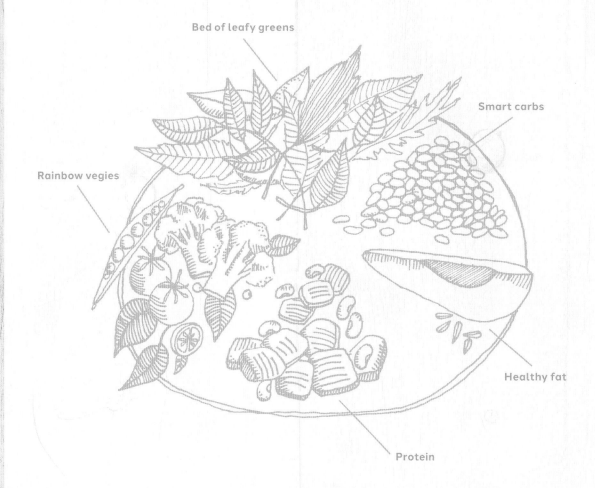

Bed of leafy greens

Smart carbs

Rainbow vegies

Healthy fat

Protein

Step 1

Get smart carbohydrates: add a fistful of slow-burning carbs for long-lasting energy and satiating appetite

Choose wholegrains over processed options. You can add precooked whole grains or starchy vegetables from your meal prepping. My favourites include sweet potato, pumpkin (squash), chickpeas (garbanzo beans), lentils, black beans, brown rice, corn, quinoa and freekeh.

Step 2

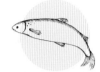

Plus a serve of lean protein

Add a serve of protein the size of your palm, or about 100–150 g (3½–5½ oz). I like to use free-range and sustainable options. Adding protein can help stabilise your blood-sugar levels, which means fewer mood swings, more stable hormones and longer-lasting fullness. Don't forget about plant-based protein options, such as legumes, nuts and seeds, or tofu. My favourites include salmon, locally caught white fish, chicken, 2 eggs, half a cup of legumes, a handful of nuts, 100 g (3½ oz) of tofu, half a cup of ricotta or cottage cheese or lean red meat.

Step 3

Throw in 'healthy' fats

Don't skip the fats! They will help you stay fuller for longer. Adding fat will also help you enjoy healthy eating more so it won't feel like a chore. My favourite fats include a quarter of an avocado, a handful of seeds and nuts, 30 g (1 oz) cheese such as feta, or dips like pesto, hummus and tahini (about 1–2 tablespoons).

Step 4

Add leafy greens and a rainbow of coloured vegetables

The more colours, the better. Put 2–3 cups of leafy greens on your plate. My favourite greens include rocket (arugula), baby spinach, cos (romaine) lettuce, mixed leaves or kale. Be sure to add colourful vegetables for beautiful antioxidants. Any colourful veg is great. Some ideas are: cherry tomatoes, shredded coleslaw mix, shredded carrots, red onion, cooked asparagus, zucchini (courgette) or capsicum (pepper) and baked vegetables.

Step 5

Add flavour

When healthy food tastes good, you're more likely to eat it. Include 1-2 tablespoons of a delicious dressing or sauce to finish your balanced plate. Fresh herbs are also a great way to add more flavour.

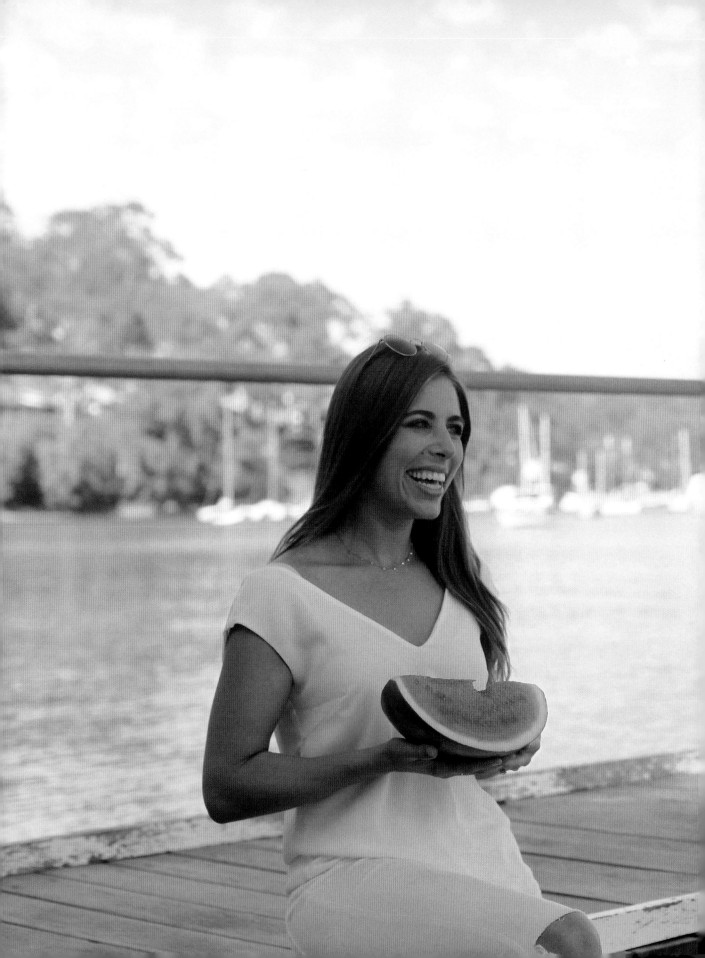

A healthy environment: how to reduce waste

Be kind to your body and be kind to the environment. Here are some tips if you're like me and love food, but hate waste.

- Always take bags with you to the grocery shops. I have a couple of cooler bags for cold things and cute hessian bags that I adore.
- Reuse jars from peanut butter, pickles and juice. Store your nuts in them or use them as a lunch box.
- Don't waste food. Order less when you eat out and take leftovers home with you. About 25 per cent of food in developed countries goes to waste! When vegies go soft, make a soup, dip or vegetable stock. Store fruit and veg properly to get the most out of shelf life.
- Cook lunch and take a lunchbox to work.
- Buy from a bulk food store. You'll save plenty of money and use far less plastic packaging.
- Don't use plastic bags when you're shopping in the produce section. Most produce doesn't need to be wrapped. Buying apples? Just put the apples directly into your shopping trolley or get reusable mesh bags.
- Keep a water bottle with you (get one you love) and you won't need plastic bottles.
- Use beeswax fabric covers instead of plastic wrap. They're reusable and sustainable.
- Wash out plastic sandwich and snack bags and hang them up to dry.
- Say 'no thanks' to single-use plastic straws.

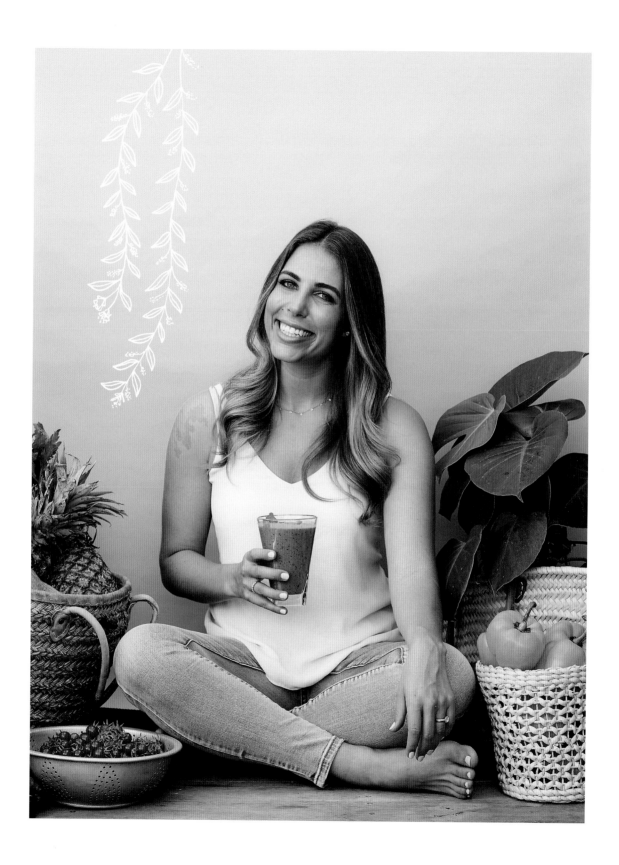

5

Heal your
relationship
with food

Your relationship with food is one of the most important you'll ever have. It doesn't matter how many years you've been struggling with this; it's never too late to make peace. It may be hard, but it's so worth it. Healing your relationship with food may be one of the best things you ever do for yourself.

Without a doubt, healing my relationship with food changed my life. In this chapter, I'm going to share some of the essential strategies for developing healthy interactions with food so you can eat with confidence, stop obsessing and keep it real.

Let me start by saying that your relationship with food is everything. A healthy diet and exercise are essential to living a good life and feeling amazing. In fact, what you eat is less important than why you eat it. By improving your relationship with food, you'll be able to choose better-for-you options more easily, without feeling the need to always control what you should or shouldn't be eating.

An unhealthy relationship with food kills motivation and sucks the joy out of eating, making it impossible to eat nutritiously and maintain a healthy weight.

Having a healthy relationship with food sets you up to naturally enjoy eating. You can break free from needing to control what you eat and obsessing about it. When you have a healthy relationship with food, it's easy to navigate Christmas time, holidays, travel, business and life and find balance with food and exercise.

Emotional eating

When I talk about emotional eating, I'm referring to eating when you aren't hungry. It can often feel out control and you feel guilty afterwards, wondering, 'why did I do that?' Even if you aren't binge eating every day, almost everyone experiences some degree of emotional eating. Why does this happen?

Food is linked with your emotions, biologically and through experience. As a child, you were probably taught to finish everything on your plate (instead of listening to your hunger), and perhaps you were rewarded with treat foods and disciplined by not getting to have dessert. Now that you're an adult, you celebrate birthdays and parties with food and even mourn sad occasions with food; your social life revolves around food—meeting friends for breakfast, brunch, lunch, coffee, cocktails or drinks, tea, dinner or dessert. This is reinforced by the fact that eating high fat and high sugar foods releases brain chemicals (serotonin) that make you feel good!

As you grew up, perhaps you tried to lose weight through dietary restrictions and counting calories. So your emotional connection to food grew even stronger and more complicated. Now, you may use food (and alcohol) to alter your feelings, pull you out of boredom and help you celebrate. Throw in dieting culture, diet rules, superslim and photoshopped models and it's a wonder anyone has a healthy relationship with food!

As a parent, you can help raise your children to have a healthy relationship with food (more on this on page 97) and, as an adult, no matter how toxic your relationship is with food, you can choose to make it stronger and healthier. Creating a healthy relationship with food doesn't happen overnight, especially if you've always had a messy, confusing or complicated relationship with food, but it's so incredibly worth investing in.

Just as you can't expect to speak a language fluently after only a few weeks, or even a few months, you can't expect to completely heal your relationship with food within a short time. As you proceed from novice through to intermediate, you'll notice that even though you 'mess up', it happens less often or your slip-ups or binges become less intense. Perhaps you eat less or they don't last as long.

Take note of the small wins. The small wins are progress and really do make a massive difference in the long term.

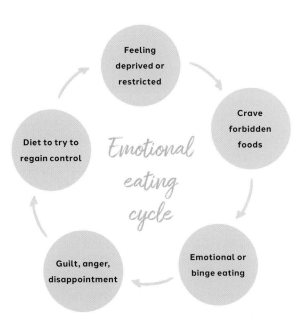

The emotional eating cycle is a set of behaviours that typically have a flow-on effect. Unless you break the cycle, you're likely to stay stuck going around and around. Ironically, many of the things you may be doing to prevent emotional eating and weight gain are having the exact opposite effect. Changing habits will help you interrupt and break free from the cycle.

HAVING AN UNHEALTHY RELATIONSHIP WITH FOOD MEANS THAT YOU:

• Lie in bed at night worrying about what you've eaten that day
• Plan meals far in advance
• Fear certain foods or food groups
• Feel judged by others when you eat
• Judge others on what they are eating or the shape of their bodies
• Think of food as either good or bad
• Worry that there isn't enough food
• Consider getting seconds before you've finished your first serving
• Subscribe to diet rules

HAVING A HEALTHY RELATIONSHIP WITH FOOD MEANS THAT YOU:

• Eat when you're hungry and stop when you're full
• Never feel deprived or restricted
• Aren't obsessed with food
• Don't feel guilt when you overeat or enjoy your favourite food
• Feel relaxed when ordering at restaurants, choosing from buffets, travelling or socialising
• Trust that there will always be more
• Don't subscribe to any diet rules
• Trust your body to guide you to a healthy weight

Disrupt the emotional eating cycle

Identify which stage of the cycle you're at and try these strategies to break free.

Stage 1. Diet to try to regain control

Resist the temptation to undereat, diet or restrict your food intake. Undereating will not 'balance out' your overeating. It will cause feelings of deprivation and, probably, more out-of-control eating. Eat 'normally' instead, listening to your hunger and appetite. Give yourself permission to eat when you're hungry.

Stage 2. Feeling deprived or restricted

When you're feeling deprived and restricted you use words like, 'I'm not allowed…', 'I shouldn't…' or 'I'm trying to be good'. Give yourself permission to eat. You may need to eat slightly more during the day (for example, have a sandwich instead of a salad) so that you feel satiated and not deprived.

Stage 3. Crave forbidden foods

Give yourself permission to eat forbidden foods in public. Order pasta at a restaurant, get peanut butter on toast at a café or buy a hot chocolate instead of a coffee. Don't create lists of 'bad' food. Practise 'crowding' by filling up on more nutritious foods.

Stage 4. Emotional or binge eating

Accept that it happened. Let go of the guilt as this will keep you stuck in the cycle. Become aware of the thoughts you're having when you are emotional eating. By being 'present' during a binge and curious, instead of angry or disappointed, you can identify exactly what triggered the binge, helping you prevent future episodes.

THE DIFFERENCE BETWEEN EMOTIONAL AND PHYSICAL HUNGER

Sometimes, you end up eating when you are 'emotionally' hungry, as opposed to physically hungry. It helps to know the difference between the two. Ask yourself: What does physical hunger feel like for me? What does emotional hunger feel like for me?

Stage 5. Feel guilt, anger and disappointment

See each time you overeat as an opportunity to learn more about yourself. Ask yourself: why did it happen and what can I do next time? Let go of the food guilt. Feeling angry and beating yourself up will likely trigger another binge and won't help you eat less next time. Accept that it is not something to be ashamed about. Don't blame yourself.

Stop relying on willpower

Have you ever said to yourself, 'If only I had more willpower or self-control, I'd be able to lose the weight'? Most people expect their willpower and self-control to help them eat better, but that's a massive mistake because your willpower is incredibly unreliable. Research published in the *Psychological Bulletin* of the American Psychological Association[1] has suggested that willpower isn't like a muscle that gets stronger with use, but rather it becomes depleted. Willpower is a limited resource. If you use it all up trying to control everything that goes into your mouth all week, you may run out of steam by the weekend.

This is another reason why diet rules don't work. You don't have an unlimited supply of self-control, so you must be stingy with how

Physical hunger	Emotional hunger
Comes on gradually and can be postponed	Comes on urgently and suddenly
Can be satisfied with any type of food e.g. apple or broccoli	Causes specific cravings such as bread, pasta, chocolate
Once you're full, you can stop eating	You eat more than you normally would. You feel uncomfortably full
You feel satisfied, not guilty, after eating	You feel guilty and angry after eating

you spend it. Willpower is like a fair-weather friend, only supporting you when things are going well. You need to be well rested, stress-free and well fed at all times, or willpower will leave you faster than you can get a tub of ice cream from the freezer.

Willpower only works when there are no other distractions, but life is unpredictable. You can't control everything that happens, which is what willpower demands of you. If you want to be healthy, you need more than just willpower to keep you motivated. Once you accept that willpower can't be relied upon, you can start to implement other strategies that will actually work, no matter how vulnerable you get. This is how you keep it real.

Here are some things to do instead of relying on willpower.

Don't watch TV while you eat

Do you eat in front of the TV (or at your desk in front of the computer screen)? I'm not going to sugar-coat things here. If you eat and watch TV simultaneously, you will almost always overeat. Why? It's called conditioning. Eating in front of the TV programs your brain to expect food when you turn on the screen. Once conditioned, turning on the TV will prompt your body to release a bunch of hunger hormones telling your brain it's time to eat, even if you weren't hungry before. Once you start eating, it's much harder to stop. Because

you're tuned into the Kardashians (or David Attenborough) and not tuned into your body, you eat mindlessly.

I used to be a TV watching binge-eater. I'd eat well all day until I got home and then, with no willpower left, I'd eat in front of the TV. I just kept eating and then I'd feel so guilty afterwards. Just like me, you too can break the habit: you don't need to give up watching TV, simply make the decision not to eat at the same time. So, if you're watching a show and feel hungry, press pause, go to the kitchen, eat at the table and then come back to finish watching the program. I understand this is a really hard habit to break, but making this one change can have incredible results.

Bring it back to basics

Feeling off balance with your health? Overwhelmed or confused? Bring it back to basics and just focus on the fundamentals. There really are so many things you COULD be doing to be healthier and feel more amazing. But heck, life is full on! To be honest, there are only so many s%*ts to give in a day so you have to be fussy about how you give them out because 'having it all' isn't possible. You've got to keep it real. So instead of fussing over things that don't fundamentally 'move the dial', focus your attention on the 20 per cent of habits that make 80 per cent of the difference to your health. Giving your

There are no 'good' or 'bad' foods: all food is neutral. When you attach these labels to food, it becomes emotionally charged. Remember, all food can play a part in a healthy diet.

attention to the things that'll make the biggest impact can save you time, energy and may even help prevent a mental breakdown.

Before addressing other areas of health, prioritise your mental energy to check off these key fundamentals. The 'nice-to-haves'—hundreds of small changes you can make—are still great to adopt once you feel comfortable with the 'fundamentals'.

These habits make 80 per cent of the difference:

- Get seven to nine hours of sleep
- Eat five to six serves of vegetables a day
- Eat two serves of fruit
- Connect with friends and family regularly; have a laugh
- Manage your stress (meditate, see a counsellor or psychologist, call a friend, keep a journal, take time off, say no, make a change)
- Cook at home
- Move your body several times a week in an enjoyable manner
- Don't drink too much alcohol
- Don't smoke or do drugs
- Drink enough water

Change your food language

The language you use can have a powerful impact on your relationship with food by adding an emotional charge to it, either demonising it or giving it 'holy' status. Changing the language you use about food is a subtle yet powerful way to drastically improve your relationship.

Using words like 'bad' or 'nasties' is judgmental and can lead to guilt and shame. For example, if you label cake as a 'bad' food, any time you eat a piece of cake you're going to feel guilty because you hold judgements that it is wrong to eat cake. But having a delicious piece of cake can be part of a healthy diet, especially as birthday cake is such a normal part of life celebrations. Making a rule that you can never have cake isn't healthy or balanced. It'll put you on the fast track to deprivation and emotional eating.

Be cautious when you see wellness bloggers or 'experts' referring to 'bad' food, 'nasties', toxic ingredients, or advising you to limit, avoid or cut out foods. This extreme and restrictive language is very unhealthy for your relationship with food.

HERE ARE SOME EASY WORDS TO SWAP:

Bad food ◄ - - ► Sometimes food
Good food ◄ - - ► Everyday food
Avoid or limit ◄ - - ► Swap

heal your relationship with food

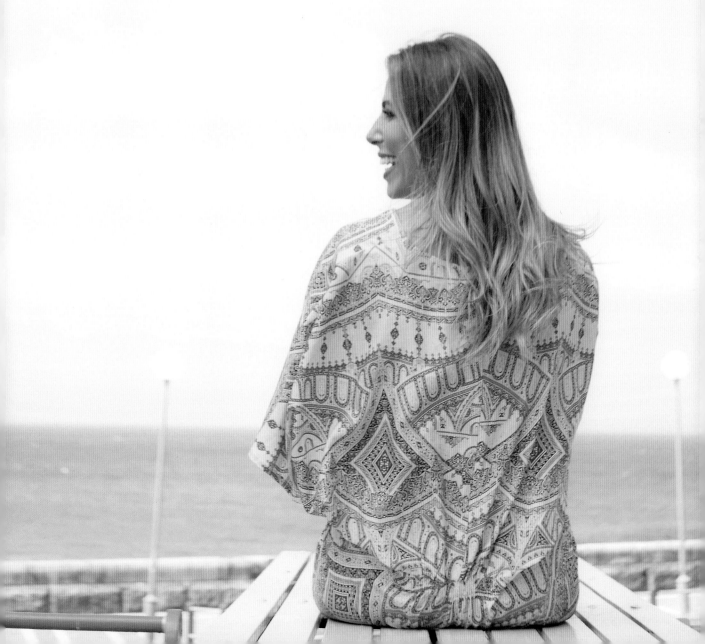

language can have
a powerful impact

EVERYDAY FOODS

Fill your diet with these 'everyday' foods. You'll naturally crowd out the 'sometimes' foods by filling up on these fresh options.

• Home-cooked food
• Vegetables: in salads, or baked and grilled
• Fresh or frozen fruit
• Seeds and nuts, all types
• Legumes and beans
• Lean protein: eggs, fish, chicken, turkey
• 'Healthy' fats: avocado, extra virgin olive oil, tahini
• Dairy foods: plain Greek-style yoghurt, milk, cheese
• Unprocessed wholegrains: barley, brown rice, buckwheat, freekeh, oats, quinoa, spelt
• Sourdough, brown and wholegrain breads

SOMETIMES FOODS

You don't need to eliminate these foods altogether. Give yourself permission to enjoy these 'sometimes' foods ... sometimes!

• Ready-made meals: takeaway (takeout), commercially prepared frozen meals
• Red meat (eat <350 g per week)
• Alcohol
• Refined bread and grains
• Sugary and refined cereals
• Ice cream, pudding, lollies (candy or sweets)
• Commercially baked goods: cake, pastries, biscuits, muffins
• Fried foods: chips, schnitzel, moneybags, spring rolls
• Fast food: burgers, pizza
• Juice, soft drinks (soda) including diet drinks, mixers and cordial
• Processed deli meat: sausages, bacon, prosciutto, chorizo, salami

Everyday and sometimes foods

Everyday foods and sometimes foods are a far healthier way to refer to 'good' or 'bad' food, because sometimes it's healthy to have a treat but every day it's best to fill up on healthier food. 'Everyday foods' are the nutritious ingredients we want to eat every day: fruit, vegetables, wholegrains, nuts, seeds, lean protein, 'good' fats and dairy. 'Sometimes foods' are foods that we should aim to eat less often, such as alcohol, chocolate, ice cream, lollies (candy or sweets), chips, pizza, soft drink (soda) and so on.

Referring to 'sometimes' and 'everyday' food feeling too restrictive for you? No problem. Food is food! Let go of the labels all together and just embrace eating intuitively.

Give yourself permission

As long as you have a list of forbidden foods, you will be likely to crave them and feel deprived. Feeling restricted often leads to obsession, guilt and emotional eating. It may feel counterintuitive (and scary!) to give yourself permission to eat the foods you've been denying yourself for all these years.

When I first reintroduced carbs to my diet, I was scared that I'd regain weight, but I didn't. When I gave myself permission to eat dessert again, my weight remained the same. In fact, lifting my restrictions and letting myself enjoy everything in moderation helped me feel in control around food again.

Keep it real: no single food or ingredient can make or break your diet. It's the big picture that counts.

As you know, the minute you make something off limits, it becomes infinitely more desirable. When you give yourself permission to eat those foods again, you remove the scarcity mindset that keeps you thinking, 'I've ruined it now, I may as well finish the whole block'. You begin to trust that any time you want more, you can have it. Food will not be withheld or taken away from you (as in a diet!). So you begin to change: you tell yourself, 'I am allowed to eat this food any time I want, but I don't really want any more right now.'

Giving yourself permission is incredibly important. You can't skip this step.

Reintroducing previously 'forbidden' foods

Here are some suggestions to help you find more balance in your diet. Eating this way will help you stabilise your blood-sugar levels, hormones and mood.

Step 1. Include 'forbidden' foods in meals.

You often binge on trigger foods during an emotional eating episode, but then avoid them when you're trying to be good. Now it's time to include them in your usual routine so you can normalise them. If you normally binge on bread, make a sandwich for lunch at work instead of having it as a snack after work while watching TV (this can be a high-risk time).

Love to eat peanut butter or chocolate hazelnut spread from the jar? Order your favourite spread on toast at a café for breakfast. Extra points if you're with someone else (see step 2).

Step 2. Make it public.

Rather than keeping your 'forbidden' foods in the house, start by eating these foods in public, with friends. This is especially important in the beginning as you start to shift out of the scarcity mindset. If you never allow yourself to eat ice cream, make plans with a friend and go out for ice cream, rather

Case study

Carly

I've been denying myself so many foods for so long. My list of forbidden foods is extensive. While I want to stop emotional eating, I am really worried that if I start eating these foods again my weight is going to spiral out of control! I avoid these foods to manage my weight. Surely if I eat them again, I'll gain heaps? I'm also scared that once I start, I won't be able to stop! Help! I'm scared and unsure.

It's perfectly normal to feel scared after avoiding these foods for so many years. Once you reintroduce these foods and give yourself permission to eat everything in moderation, the 'forbidden' foods will start to lose their power over you. One day you may be the person who pushes their dessert plate away halfway through because they're satisfied.

This is all possible when you stop restricting and truly give yourself permission to eat these foods, without fear that they will be taken away again shortly, come the next diet.

When reintroducing forbidden foods, repeat to yourself: 'I am allowed to eat this food. I can always have more when I want.' This will help you get out of the scarcity mindset (the belief that 'I have to eat it all now because I can't eat it later'). When you truly understand that you can always have more if you want to, then you will feel in control around these foods again.

Trust this process. Although it takes time, it really does work and it's worth it.

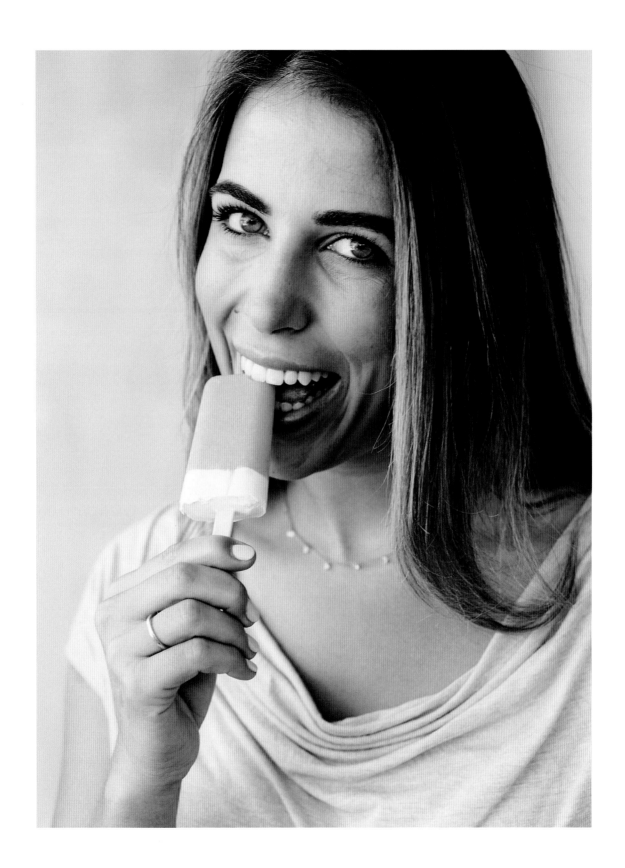

than buying a tub to keep at home. This is especially important if you're a secret eater. Out for dinner with friends? Order dessert at the restaurant instead of going home feeling that you weren't allowed. Go to an Italian restaurant and order what you really feel like eating, not just the salad or grilled fish.

Step 3. Fully enjoy the process.

Fully embrace the enjoyment of eating and don't let guilt creep into your mind. You are allowed to eat this food right now. Fully experience the taste and flavours. Chew thoroughly and let the flavour linger. Practise eating slowly, chewing thoroughly and enjoy.

Step 4. Focus on how you feel.

If you've been avoiding a food for a long time, you might not really taste it any more, especially when you binge. So take time to get to know this food again. Is it sweeter or saltier than you remember? Is it more delicious or less delicious? Do you enjoy it as much as you remember? Sometimes 'forbidden' foods can seem better in our minds. Once you really taste them, you might realise they aren't as incredible as you remember. When you recognise this, they begin to lose power.

Case study

Sophie

I love the idea that food is neither good nor bad! I know I don't feel good eating some kinds of food, but a part of me is saying, 'eat this because your parents never let you eat this stuff.' I think that, because I wasn't allowed sweets much as a kid, I naturally want more of these foods.

I am still eating fruits and vegetables and exercising every day, but I think that control is my biggest issue when that kind of food is in front of me. It's almost as though I have this idea that there is a scarcity and I will never get it, so I have to eat it all. Does this seem outrageous and strange?

This doesn't sound strange at all! In fact, very often parents unintentionally set their children up for really challenging relationships with food. I'm so glad you're aware that the 'scarcity mindset' is affecting you. This has been ingrained since you were young, so it will take time to retrain your brain. The most important thing to do is give yourself permission to eat those foods you always considered 'bad'.

You need to reteach your brain that actually, you are allowed. Over time, you'll notice that you'll be less tempted by these foods because there will be an underlying understanding that any time you really want to eat them, you're allowed to. You'll find you won't binge on these foods anymore. You may realise you don't even like them as much!

EAT WHAT YOU REALLY FEEL LIKE, MINDFULLY: *no guilt needed*

Case study

Judy

I've already started using everyday and sometimes food instead of good and bad. Wow! I didn't realise how often I used those words. I am a little confused though, as I like to have a couple of squares of chocolate every night. Technically, chocolate is a sometimes food, not an everyday food. Am I doing the wrong thing? Please don't tell me I can't have chocolate anymore!

As a fellow chocolate lover, I would never want you to deprive yourself of your favourite ritual! You're right: chocolate isn't technically an 'everyday' food but using those words is not a rule, simply a guide. It sounds like having a couple of squares of chocolate is a really balanced, healthy ritual in your life that probably prevents you from feeling like you're missing out. Even though you're having chocolate every day, you're eating small amounts. I don't think there is anything wrong with having a little chocolate every night.

If you notice that other 'sometimes' foods are sneaking into your diet every day, think about swapping them for some better-for-you options. Here are some ideas.

Swap this		for this
Salty chips	←--→	Pretzels, popcorn, nuts, seaweed snacks, roasted chickpeas, edamame
Lollies (candy or sweets)	←--→	Frozen grapes, berries, fruit
Ice cream	←--→	Yoghurt with honey, frozen banana 'ice cream'
Soft drink (soda)	←--→	Coconut water, water with mint
Banana bread	←--→	Raisin toast or mashed banana on toast
Fried foods	←--→	Baked, grilled or barbecued options

That said, sometimes a healthier swap just won't do! In which case, eat what you really feel like, mindfully: no guilt needed.

Identify your triggers

There are a number of things that commonly trigger emotional and binge eating episodes. As soon as you become aware of the things that trigger you to overeat, you become empowered and can regain control over your eating. Use the list below to tick off the triggers that resonate with you.

When I was binge eating, being home alone, feeling tired or sad, TV watching and judgmental comments were particularly triggering for me. Once I understood that certain triggers caused my emotional eating, I was empowered because I had awareness. I could predict emotional eating or understand why it had happened. It started to make sense. I made a few changes that helped me be less vulnerable.

Firstly, I started studying from the library instead of at home alone and that sure helped! I committed to no longer watching TV while eating (such a hard habit to break, but so worth it) and I spoke to the people in my life who were making triggering statements about my food and weight (see pages 108–109 for guidance on how to do this). I started seeing a counsellor so I stopped using food to numb myself, and I prioritised sleep.

Now it's your turn. Which emotional eating triggers affect you? Use the guide on page 90 to help you reduce the effects.

Help! I binge on healthy foods too!

Many people binge on 'healthy' (or 'normal') foods like peanut butter, nuts, bread and cereal. It's tough to remove these from the house completely, especially when there are other family members who love to eat them.

Even though you understand consciously that peanut butters, nuts, cereal and bread aren't 'bad' for you, that they contain lots of beneficial nutrients, these foods are often considered 'bad' in the dieting world because they contain higher amounts of energy or carbohydrates.

Tip

While reintroducing 'forbidden' foods, maintaining a healthy environment at home can help prevent a binge. Fill your house with plenty of fresh and better-for-you options and wait to feel in control around these foods again before buying them for home. There are tips on pages 64–67 to help you support healthier habits.

Give yourself permission to have your trigger foods as part of a meal: have peanut butter on toast for breakfast; eat a bowl of cereal for breakfast; have a sandwich for lunch; or add nuts to your salad or smoothie. Reintroducing these foods helps you realise that they are not forbidden or 'bad'.

A note about nuts

A handful of nuts is a really healthy snack or addition to a meal. Your body loves the 'healthy' fats, fibre and protein packed in these nutritious superfoods. But often, it's really hard to stop at one handful. Personally, one handful of nuts has never left me feeling full or satisfied. That's why I prefer to snack on fruit when I'm hungry, as I need to chew more for my brain to understand that I've eaten a meal, so I'm more mindful of the snack and feel more satisfied afterwards. I like to add nuts to my meals, such as muesli, salads and stir-fries.

Actionable strategies

Being home alone
Give yourself permission to eat in front of others, especially the foods you've always considered 'bad'. This will normalise 'forbidden' foods so they lose power over you.

Feeling tired, exhausted or sleep deprived
Reassess your sleep. Aim for 30 minutes extra sleep each night. Monitor your sleep quality with a sleep app. Buy an alarm clock. Don't sleep with your phone next to your bed. Read a book before bed to avoid the blue light from electronic devices, which has been shown to stimulate wakefulness. Wake up at the same time each morning.

Scrolling on social media
Unfollow social media accounts that make you feel bad about yourself. Unfollow accounts that you find triggering. Track your social media use with an app. Reduce social media time by 50 per cent. Stop looking for images using the 'explore' section.

When someone loses weight
Did they do it sustainably and healthily? Would their approach really work for you? Would you be willing to eat like that for the rest of your life? If not, remind yourself that you are on a long-term journey and have given up yo-yo dieting. Resist the temptation.

Feeling stressed, anxious or overwhelmed
Stop referring to food as 'good' or 'bad'. Keep listening to your hunger. Make an appointment with a counsellor or psychologist to explore your feelings. Ask people for help if you feel overrun. Practise saying no to lighten your load! Practise being kind to yourself.

Feeling happy
Think of other ways to treat yourself when things go well. Instead of getting a cocktail or cake, go to a movie, call a friend or buy a new book. Make an appointment with a counsellor or psychologist to explore your feelings.

Feeling bored
Acknowledge that you are feeling bored and that is why you are getting something to eat. Ask yourself: 'Am I hungry?' Wait until you're hungry to eat.

Watching TV
Don't eat in front of the TV. Turn off the TV to get a snack and then turn it on again once you've finished eating. This is a crucial habit to break! Drink tea or a glass of water instead.

Hearing judgmental comments about my weight or body
Have the hard conversation. Explain that the comments make it harder for you to lose weight, eat less. They are demotivating. Have no tolerance for body bullies. See page 107.

When I feel someone is judging me, my body or what I'm eating
What someone else thinks about you, your food and your body doesn't matter because they don't know the journey you have been on. Your health cannot be defined by a number on the BMI chart. Feel confident that what you are doing or eating right now is exactly right for you right now. Trust your journey.

Mel

My problem is the weekends! I actually eat really healthily during the week but then I always overindulge on the weekends. I feel like I'm undoing all the good I did during the week. Every Monday, I have to start again from scratch. It's so frustrating! It's also the same thing when I go on holidays. I'm fine when I have a routine but then I go bonkers when I have wriggle room. What can I do differently to break this pattern?

It's natural and normal to eat more indulgently on the weekend. It is typically easier to eat healthily during the week because there is more routine. First, if you feel deprived by the time you get to the weekend, then you will end up overindulging on the weekend because you finally feel like you're 'allowed'. The scarcity mindset can take over and you think, 'Well, I've ruined it now—I don't know when I'll next be allowed to eat this—so I may as well keep eating and start again tomorrow.' Start by working on reducing your guilt. You might want to give yourself permission to be more relaxed with eating on the weekend.

Second, I'd also recommend reassessing your weekend plans. If you have multiple social occasions centred around eating and drinking, then you'll probably indulge simply because of your environment. Try to socialise with friends by going for a walk, going to a movie or a show or meeting up at the beach. If you want to drink less alcohol, then make arrangements with friends earlier in the day (for breakfast or brunch), which are less likely to turn into drinking affairs! If you find you're simply doing too much on the weekend, practise saying no and fitting in more down time.

Lastly, try to use the lack of routine on the weekend and holidays to your advantage. As there are no set meal times, it's a chance to practise intuitive eating. Let go of the need to eat at usual meal times. This might mean you wait to eat until a brunch date, or have a light snack in the afternoon before going out for dinner. You may find you eat more indulgently, but you eat less in total and this balances out.

The weekend is a great time to catch up on exercise as you have more time to spare. Reserve some time to do a walk with a friend or partner, even if you grab a coffee and the paper on the way. It's a great excuse to squeeze in a bit of movement as well as down time.

Chelsea

I've noticed that when I am about to get my period, I can't stop eating, mostly all the 'wrong' foods. The cravings are strong. Is there a way you can overcome this?

Spot on: your hormones are going to bump up cravings to a big degree during this time, typically a few days before your period. While these cravings are a hard-wired biological response to changes in your hormones, there are a few things you can try.

Eat more fibre and choose options containing 'healthy' fats. These foods can increase oestrogen levels, helping you feel full and satiated and reducing sugar cravings. Foods such as nuts and seeds, avocado, full-fat dairy and wholegrains are great choices.

Track your period so you can be prepared.

Give yourself permission to eat more slow-burning, unrefined carbohydrates during this time; try a sandwich for lunch, fruit for snacks, muesli for breakfast and snacks like two to three fresh dates. You're going to crave the sugar so you may as well get it from somewhere healthy. Fruit is the perfect sweet snack, complete with slow-burning satiating fibre and plenty of antioxidants. Buy more fresh, delicious fruit and you'll mostly likely end up eating more.

Create a healthy environment at home so it makes healthy eating easier.

Sleep more and be a little more... selfish. Make time for you and prioritise sleep. Do less, organise more downtime and practise saying 'no thank you'.

Try a chocolate chia pudding or banana ice cream. Enjoy fully, without guilt. If that doesn't hit the spot, then accept that some of your favourite chocolate is what you really need. And that's perfectly OK, too.

Check in before eating

Feeling a deep desire to eat and eat... and eat? Stop and check in with what is happening for you. Before eating, try to understand what underlying emotions are driving you to feel the need to eat. When I'm feeling ashamed, guilty or anxious, I can be drawn to eat richer foods, in larger amounts. As long as I ignore these feelings, it can be tough to really tune into my appetite. By asking myself, 'What are you feeling? What is driving you to eat more?' I can get to the cause of the cravings and tackle them head on.

Reducing food guilt

I used to beat myself up for hours after eating more than I had planned to eat. Then I'd lie in bed berating myself for being such a failure. I thought beating myself up afterwards would motivate me to eat less the next day. But in fact, my food guilt kept me stuck in the emotional eating cycle (see page 79). When I was on a 'health kick' (the socially acceptable way of restricting), I'd feel guilty from deviating, even slightly, if I had a bite of a dessert or ate an extra piece of fruit. As long as I was dieting, I felt guilty for not being perfect. These days, when I have dessert or eat a little too much, I don't feel guilty about it. Not even a little bit guilty! Why? Because I realised that a guilt trip doesn't help. I decided that life is too short to obsess over carbohydrates or feel guilty for eating cake. If even a hint of guilt arises, I acknowledge it and then gently push it out my mind. My mental wellbeing is more important than having a 'perfect' body.

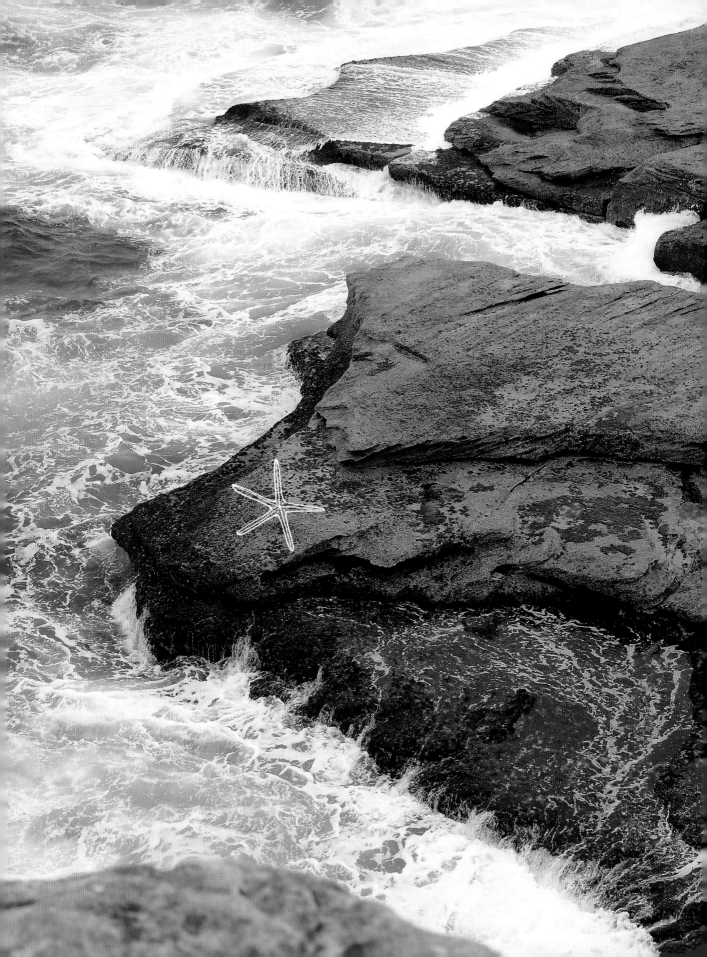

INDULGENCES ARE A PART OF A *balanced diet*

Why does food guilt happen?

Notice how you only feel guilty after eating 'bad' food? You will feel guilty when your expectation of what you think you 'should' be doing does not align with the reality. For example, 'I shouldn't have had a piece of cake' or 'I didn't need to drink that much'. When you eat what you think is the 'wrong' food or too much food, you start to beat yourself up and give yourself a hard time, hoping that it'll motivate you to eat less next time. The problem is that guilt causes the exact opposite to happen. Feeling guilty after eating drives emotional eating. Food guilt makes you eat more (not less) because:

- It emotionally supercharges food. Instead of seeing chocolate as 'neutral', it's labeled good or bad. So when you've had a bad day, you tell yourself you deserve the chocolate. If chocolate was 'neutral', then you wouldn't use it as a reward as much.
- It motivates you to restrict (aka diet), keeping you stuck in the emotional eating cycle. Even if you overeat, if you can stop feeling guilty, you can break free from the emotional eating cycle.
- Reprimanding yourself about what you have eaten makes you think about it more, not less, making it easy to obsess and stress about food. The less you think and worry about food, the easier it is to get on with your life and eat intuitively.
- It encourages black-and-white-thinking. You may think, 'well, I've ruined it already, I may as well finish the block of chocolate'. If you didn't feel guilty for eating some chocolate,

you'd be more likely to feel content after a few pieces. 'I was allowed to eat the chocolate. It was delicious and yummy. I feel like I've had enough now. I know I can always have more when I want.'

- It can make you fear foods, which can lead to extreme, obsessive and unhealthy habits. Food guilt gets worse over time, so you begin to feel guilty for eating a piece of bread when a little while ago you ate a sandwich without a worry. Food guilt makes you fear more foods.
- It can derail your efforts. One slip up does not ruin your diet. But food guilt can convince you otherwise. When you aren't affected by food guilt, you're able to see indulgences as part of healthy eating.

Feeling guilty after eating (not overeating) is the main reason you fall off the wagon. If you can stop feeling guilty after eating, then you can start to reduce overeating and emotional eating. You can break the cycle.

How to reduce food guilt

Practise crowding by filling up on more fresh food. Don't focus on what you're not allowed to eat, simply aim to make healthy choices e.g. aim to eat more vegetables.

- Listen to your hunger. Don't restrict, just eat according to your appetite.
- Focus on how you FEEL, not what you THINK. When you finish eating, ask yourself 'how did that make me feel?' If you overeat, chances are you won't feel good. It is a much better motivator because it's a physical feeling. When you try to control what you eat, you'll

heal your relationship with food

Claire

My problem is that I mainly overeat when I get home from work. I eat so much and can't stop. By the time it gets to dinner, I'm not even hungry so I can't eat with my family. Why is that happening? What can I do about it?

After work is a really common time to overeat. It sounds like you're probably exhausted after a long day, maybe dealing with some stress AND hungry. Over time, you may have conditioned your brain to know that you'll get fed as soon as you get home.

It's time to recondition your brain. Rather than waiting to get home before you eat, I'd recommend packing a snack with you for work, such as a banana or a piece of grainy toast with avocado. Eat it just before leaving the office, if you feel hungry.

Also, check you are eating enough during the day. If you're 'trying to be good' during the day, you may be undereating. When you get home, you're so exhausted and your willpower has been depleted so you end up overeating. If you're having a salad for lunch, then maybe you need to swap to a salad sandwich instead. By giving yourself permission to have more food during the day, particularly satiating food, you probably won't be as hungry nor feel deprived.

Lastly, if you're consistently tired and stressed, then a more substantial change might be needed. Are you happy at work? Can you improve your sleep quality? Working to reduce stress and exhaustion will tackle the underlying cause.

always struggle. But when you physically don't enjoy eating like that, then you'll find it more motivating in the long term.

- Forgive yourself. If you overeat, let it go. Release the judgement about how you should eat. When you notice the judgmental voice berating you, acknowledge it and then switch the station. You won't stop feeling guilty right away. Take some time to change this. Keep working to reduce your judgement over food and eat intuitively.

- Work on your perfectionism. Food guilt happens when your expectations are incredibly high. Chances are, you're a perfectionist and you're expecting your eating to be perfect too. To let go of guilt, work on your need for perfection.

- Giving yourself permission to eat your 'forbidden' foods; eating intuitively; changing your food language from 'good' and 'bad'; and no longer rigidly controlling what you eat can also really help.

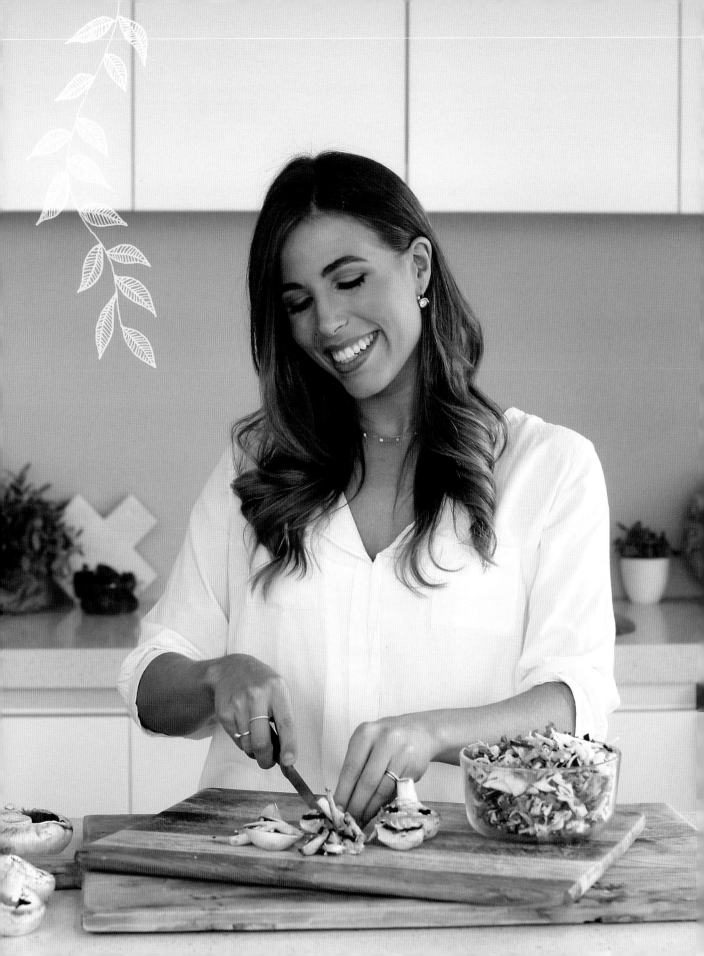

Teach your children to have a healthy relationship with food

This can set them up for a lifetime of healthy habits and prevent them feeling body conscious. Here are some key strategies to give children a balanced approach to food.

Have your own healthy relationship with food.

You're doing this already, right now, by reading this book. By embracing the principles you learn, you will be leading by example. Your children will see you enjoying a dessert, along with everyone else, exercising for enjoyment and eating bright and colourful vegetables at meals.

Update your food language.

Using healthy food language around children is crucial. Research from the University of Michigan Children's Hospital[2] has shown that mothers of obese children use different words related to eating. Parents of children with obesity problems were more likely to use direct statements such as, 'you're only allowed one more' to get their children to stop eating. Other mothers used less direct statements such as, 'you have had dinner'.

Don't refer to weight.

Never tell children that foods will make you fat or help you lose weight. Instead, talk about how food makes you feel and what it does for you. Explain how some foods give us great energy so we can do the things we love, like sports and playing, and that some foods make us feel better than others. Teach them to eat all the colours of the rainbow to get all the nutrients needed to grow strong and healthy.

Teach intuitive eating.

Remember being taught to finish everything on your plate? This advice encourages children to ignore natural hunger and appetite cues. Teach your children to tune into their hunger. Explain that hunger is telling us when we are ready to eat and fullness is our bodies' smart way of saying it's time to stop eating. If they aren't hungry, don't force them. If they want food, ask them if they are hungry or bored or tired or something else? If they really are hungry, ask them to try to describe how it feels. Let them fill up on healthy, everyday foods until they feel full.

Don't let children eat in front of the TV.

This is hard one, I know. But this habit starts as a kid and stays with you. Children who eat at the table, instead of in front of the TV or a device, are a lot more mindful of their food and are less likely to keep eating once they are full.

Resist the urge to judge yourself.

Speak kindly to yourself: your children listen closely to everything you say. Making comments about how much you hate your body or complaining when you feel fat or have overeaten teaches them that this is OK.

Resist the urge to judge others.

If you judge people by what they eat, how much they weigh, how attractive or intelligent they are, your children will notice. It teaches them to judge and compare themselves to other people. Like all of us, your children will have things they start to feel self-conscious about. They begin to think, 'If people judge that person for being overweight, "hairy" or stupid, then they will judge me too.' Teach your children to be self-assured and confident by embracing all different people.

Create a healthy environment.

If you fill the house with fresh, healthy food options, that's what your children will eat. Chores like setting the table, while helpful, don't always instil a sense of excitement about food time, so get your kids involved in meal prep and take them shopping as well. Let them choose fruit for their lunchbox. Ask them to mix a salad dressing or add the ingredients into a bowl.

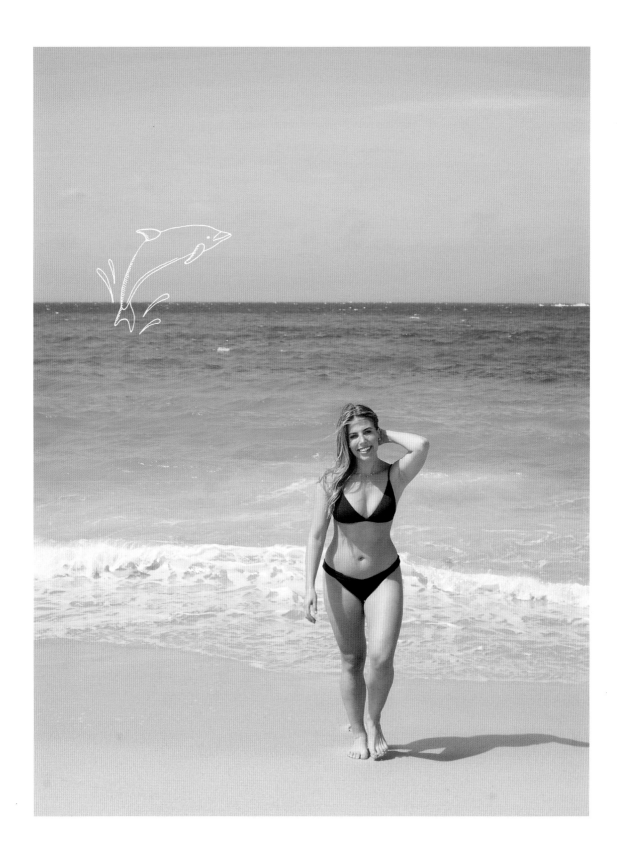

boost your *body image*

How many years have you spent wishing your body was different? If you don't want to spend the rest of your life hating your body, it's time to boost your body image. The surprising truth is that when you love your body, it's actually far easier to take care of your health and find your happiest weight.

Having poor body image never motivated me to lose weight. Instead, it made me feel self-conscious, depressed, anxious and uncomfortable and it killed my self-confidence. As long as I hated my body, I could never truly love myself.

I used to force myself to stare at my naked body in the mirror so I would be shamed into losing weight. 'If I know how truly fat and ugly I am, I'll be more motivated to lose weight,' I thought, but I was wrong. You can't shame yourself or hate your body into losing weight.

Because I felt so bad about myself, I was more vulnerable on 'bad' days. I would stop at the shops on the way home to get a bag of chocolates or chips (instead of going for a walk). Once my body image improved, I became more resilient, my anxiety reduced and I was stronger.

A healthy body image is one of the best gifts you can give yourself. When you have healthy body image:

· You take better care of yourself.
· You become less vulnerable to life's challenges.
· You may be less likely to emotionally eat after a tiring or challenging day.
· You exercise because you love your body, not as punishment for eating.
· You groom your body and make sure it's clean, energised and feeling good.
· You make time for rest, self-care and enjoyable activities.
· You have more perspective.
· You can stop suffering and hurting.
· It feels so good to not to always worry about the number on the scales.
· You have much more time in the day to do the things that make you happy because you don't waste your time worrying about not being good or thin enough.

Eating disorders

The typical image of a person with an eating disorder is someone who is skeletally thin. The thing is, you don't need to look a certain way to have an eating disorder. Eating disorders affect people of all shapes and sizes.

There are a number of eating disorders, such as anorexia nervosa, bulimia nervosa and others with less specific names. People with eating disorders have high mortality rates[1]. If you are worried that you might have an eating disorder, please visit your doctor and explain what has been happening.

Body dysmorphia

It's natural not to love every single part of your body, but when you spend hours thinking about your imperfections and flaws each day, chances are you have body dysmorphia. If someone tells you that you look good, you don't believe they're telling the truth. Even a slight imperfection or perceived flaw can feel incredibly overwhelming, as though that is all anyone is focusing on. This fear of judgement keeps you stuck, living small and feeling scared to step into who you are meant to be. Body dysmorphia can really impact on your quality of life, causing you to miss out on social occasions and opportunities because you fear not being good enough.

Looking back, I realise that I suffered from body dysmorphia for many years. And I know so many other women (and men) who will feel the same when they read the list of signs at right.

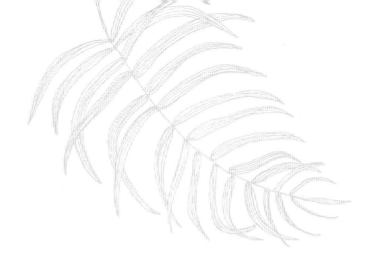

Luckily, I got help. Body Dysmorphia Disorder is a mental disorder and, if you don't treat it, it can lead to depression, anxiety and suicidal thoughts. The best thing to do is to contact your GP and get a referral to a psychologist or counsellor. I'm so glad I did.

Orthorexia

Orthorexia was recently acknowledged as a serious eating disorder, in which sufferers have an unhealthy obsession with being healthy. In the social media age, this eating disorder has taken off as fitspo (short for 'fitness inspiration') is taken to the extreme and healthy eating inspiration has turned into a set of rules to follow. While someone with anorexia nervosa may obsess about calories, those with orthorexia are obsessed with only eating foods deemed 'healthy enough'. This often results in sufferers cutting out entire food groups, or fearing foods and social occasions because healthy eating becomes challenging; going out for dinner with friends becomes a logistical nightmare.

This obsession with 'healthy' eating actually becomes really unhealthy, because it stops you from living a normal life. Food controls your thoughts and your life revolves around meals and exercise. You might feel guilty for eating anything that isn't 'good' enough. Orthorexia is a serious eating disorder. Like all eating disorders, the best treatment is to start by speaking to your doctor who can refer you to a dietitian and a psychologist for support.

SIGNS THAT YOU MAY HAVE BODY DYSMORPHIA DISORDER MAY INCLUDE:

- Trying to hide your body part under make-up, scarves, hats, clothing
- Constantly comparing yourself with others
- Seeking plastic surgery
- Constantly checking in a mirror
- Avoiding mirrors and photographs
- Picking at your skin
- Excessive grooming or exercise
- Changing clothes excessively often
- Avoiding social occasions
- Feeling anxious, depressed and ashamed
- Not trusting people when they say you look fine
- Asking other people if you look OK

Note: These are just some of the habits that can be associated with body dysmorphia. If some of them apply to you, it doesn't necessarily mean that you have the disorder. Talk to your doctor or psychologist if you are worried that you might be suffering.

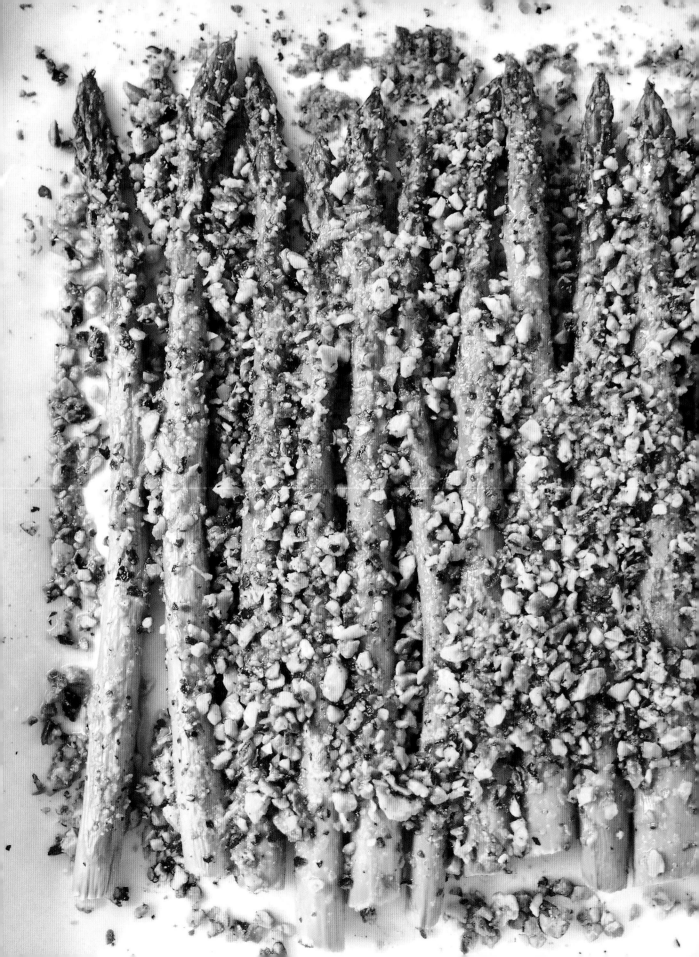

Binge-eating disorder

Binge-eating disorder or BED was only really recognised as a diagnosable eating disorder in 2013. It's a serious mental disorder with two main features: eating a very large amount of food within a relatively short period of time (for example, within two hours) and feeling a loss of control while eating (feeling unable to stop yourself). If you think you may have binge-eating disorder, contact your GP to explain your symptoms. You can get help!

In the meantime, here's some ideas of what to do immediately after you binge:

- Do not restrict or deprive yourself. Don't try to be extra 'good' to outweigh what you just ate. This may cause more emotional eating.
- Check in with your hunger. Ask yourself: 'Am I hungry?'
- See your binge or emotional eating episode as an opportunity. Learn from each binge to try and understand why you binged.
- Keep track of the days when you do not binge or eat emotionally. Look for trends in the days of the week. This is also a great way to track your progress.
- Don't aim for perfection. Just aim for progress. Be realistic with your goals.
- Be patient and kind to yourself. You can't rush recovery. It took you many years to have this relationship with food and it's going to take you a long time to heal your relationship with food.

The scarcity mindset

After years of dieting, it's very common to suffer from anxiety about 'food scarcity'; the conscious (and often subconscious) fear that there isn't enough food. Even if you can physically see the food, you don't have certainty that this abundance will always be available to you. This comes from years of restricting yourself, so when you have the chance to eat, you feel that you should eat as much as possible because you won't be 'allowed' to eat it later.

When you operate from the scarcity mindset, you don't relate to food normally because your body goes into a primal state. There is no point of satiation or control; it's 'all-or-nothing' thinking. As long as you have this mindset, you will continue to feel as if you're always eating your last meal, unsure and untrusting when you'll next be able to eat what you truly desire.

Use the following tips to break free from the scarcity mindset:

- Give yourself permission to eat the foods you want to eat. When you do, these foods will lose their power and control over you.
- Remind yourself that there is always more if you are still hungry. And then ensure that you make good on your promise. If you are hungry, you must eat. You need your body to trust that it will always be fed when hungry. This means no skipping meals.
- Practise eating slowly and mindfully and enjoy it. If you are still hungry after an hour, go and get more food.
- Eat your 'trigger' or binge foods in front of other people. Challenge trigger foods by bringing them into your everyday life.
- Stop striving for weight loss. Ironically, aiming to lose weight is keeping you stuck. Make health the focus, not weight. Invest your energy into making and keeping healthy behaviours instead of worrying about what you can or can't eat.

Trauma and grief

Many people use eating as a way to numb grief and pain. Many of my clients have experienced traumatic events such as the death of someone dear to them, the loss of a job, big life changes or emotional abuse.

If you have had a traumatic event in your past, it may still be affecting you and causing emotional eating. The best thing to do is to make an appointment with a psychologist or a counsellor who can help you work through the pain you feel. Food can only ever provide temporary relief.

Comparisons

Comparing yourself with others can be addictive, like a train wreck you can't look away from, like an itch that has to be scratched. I used to tell myself that comparing myself with others would motivate me to be better, inspire me to 'pull myself together' and become amazing. It never did. I'd compare myself with other women who I thought were doing better than me, looked better than me and seemed to have everything. At the beach, seeing a girl with the 'perfect' body or incredibly chic accessories and outfit could make me feel inferior within a second. Or I'd get stuck in a social media vortex and suddenly, I'd be scrolling through photos from a year ago, feeling self-pity and completely inadequate.

I had convinced myself that comparing myself with others would inspire me, make me better and strong. But comparison actually did the opposite. Comparison would paralyse me and envy would take hold within seconds. Instead of forging ahead with an exciting goal, I was left curled up like a ball, thinking, 'I'll never be that good, so what's the point of trying?'

Constantly comparing yourself with others can feel good at times. At some point you need to stop and decide that enough is enough. Want the good news? Comparison is a habit, and all habits can be broken. Here are a few strategies to help you overcome the need to compare yourself with others.

Smile

When you see someone in public who makes you feel envious, smile at them. I do this trick all the time. Making you feel intimidated? Smile. A big genuine smile. Most often, they will smile back at you. And instead of feeling like the outsider, you're suddenly their secret stranger friend who may have brightened up their day.

We all struggle

No matter how accomplished, beautiful or well-off you are, everyone has bad days and their own set of worries that keeps them up at night. From the outside, their life may seem glamorous, perfect and enviable, but there is a lot that you can't see from the outside or from social media. Know that you're seeing their highlights reel, not real life. Acknowledge that we all hurt from time to time. Even if you were more beautiful, more successful, it doesn't mean you'd be happier.

Be grateful

Take a moment out to be grateful for what you have. Envy doesn't exist well in the presence of gratitude. Be grateful to feel the sun on your face, to be able to breathe, to walk or to smell. Even the smallest moments of gratitude can help break the comparison trap.

Unplug and unfollow

Get really smart about how you use social media. Unfollow anyone who makes you feel envious or inferior. Disconnect from social media as much as possible. How about scaling back to once or twice a day check-ins? It sounds hard, but maybe that's a clue that it's worth trying. Stop using the 'explore' function, which can lure you into a comparison vortex.

COMPARISON IS A *habit,* AND ALL HABITS CAN BE *broken*

Self-sabotage

Chances are you're a self-saboteur and you don't realise it. Can't attain that longstanding goal? You may be self-sabotaging. Self-sabotage is when you delay achieving a certain goal (perhaps the goal feels too hard, confronting, boring) by engaging in another behaviour that ultimately distracts you from the underlying challenge. Some forms of self-sabotage include procrastination, self-medication (taking drugs, drinking alcohol, smoking) and emotional eating. Being a self-saboteur can make you feel like you're stuck, postponing the inevitable, not really dipping a toe into the unknown because it's too scary.

Are you avoiding emotions? It's much easier to push feelings aside instead of sitting down with yourself and getting to know what's aching inside. But you're really just kicking the can down the road, delaying the pain; and the longer it's left, the harder it gets. It's time to tackle those emotions.

Acknowledging you're self-sabotaging is step one. Step two is getting help.

Reduce your goals. Do you dream of exercising four to five days a week? Huge goals can be paralysing because they feel too hard and overwhelming. Break down the goal. Does exercising two or three days a week feel more doable? Give yourself a long time to accomplish your goals.

Embrace small progress. The little things really do add up to make something big happen. Reward yourself for any progress, however small. You procrastinate or avoid emotions because the short-term motivation outweighs the long-term gratification. By embracing small wins, you make the long-term game more enticing and the whole process is less daunting.

Feel the feels. As long as your feelings stay at arm's distance, you'll be in neutral, not going or coming. Feeling emotions like anger doesn't mean you'll start yelling at the convenience store clerk. In fact, by acknowledging and processing your feelings, you may be less vulnerable to emotional outbursts. A psychologist or counsellor will be able to help you work through the emotions you're avoiding.

Feeling judged: by yourself and others.

We all judge. I judge people who walk or drive too slowly in front of me. I judge people who always run late. But mostly, I judge myself. The good news? I am aware of my judgments, and this gives me power because when you have awareness, you can make a change. Noticing when you make judgments can empower you to act and think differently and this can free you from feeling guilty and judging yourself.

Judgement is another form of numbing out the feeling, avoiding emotions. We often judge others more when we are not feeling good, when we feel vulnerable and, specifically, we judge them on the things we feel vulnerable about. People who are truly content with who they are rarely feel the need to judge others.

The more judgment we receive, the more we learn how to judge. Social media is based on judgements – like or not like. Share or not share. Comment or no comment. When you notice you are being judgmental, make

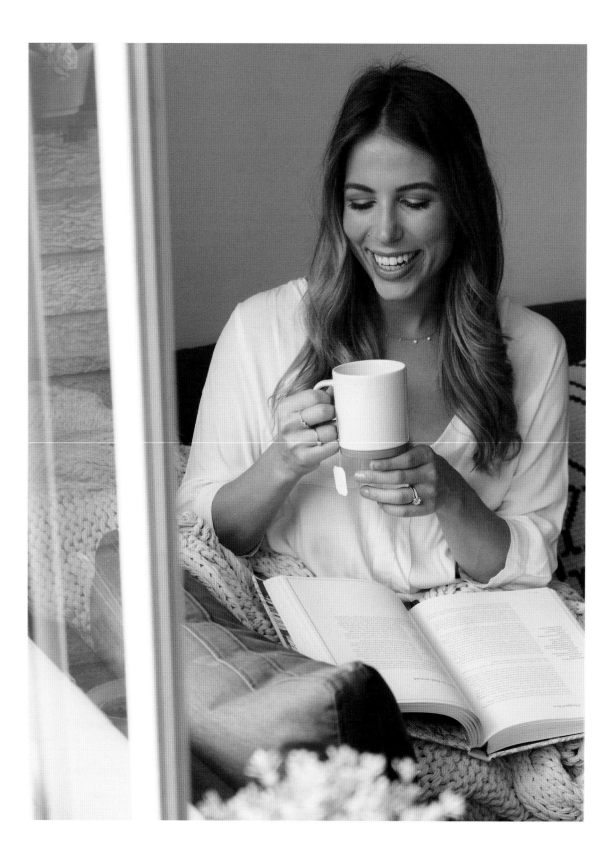

a life pivot so you can divert your energy to something else. Here are some things you can do when you notice you are judging yourself or someone else:

- Choose not to speak the judgement out loud
- Change the topic or thought
- Distract yourself (listen to some music)
- Forgive yourself
- Notice the judgment, without judging yourself for judging

Over time, you learn to care less about what other people think of you and more about what you think of yourself. As long as you give yourself a hard time, you will turn to others for validation (and will continue to feel judged). Once you accept yourself, you give yourself the validation you need. You no longer look to others for approval or validation and, as such, you no longer feel judged.

Food police and body bullies

You may not be the only one trashing your body. Sometimes, the people closest to you can be the harshest critics or trigger you the most about your body. They can assume the role of food police or body bully in an attempt to help you lose weight or fit in. Often, mothers or partners take on these roles, which can be harmful to your body image and health.

Another of my clients, Rob, explained how his doctor had body bullied him at a routine check-up. The doctor spent the whole appointment reprimanding Rob for weighing too much, even though Rob had simply made the appointment to get travel vaccinations. Instead of motivating Rob to lose weight, Rob went home and ate until he felt sick. When Rob received unsolicited advice about his weight, it triggered emotional eating.

Claire's story is similar. Desperate to finally lose weight, Claire asked her husband to help keep her accountable with her latest diet. At first she found his support helpful, but very quickly she felt judged. Claire's husband is also very conscious of his weight and judgmental of other people's bodies. He became her food police. Sentences like, 'you shouldn't be eating that, you'll get fat,' became commonplace. Claire felt judged by her husband and no longer felt she could eat 'normally' in front of him. She began to eat in secret, further adding to her guilt and shame about her body. As her weight spiralled out of control, her relationship with her husband became strained and her overeating increased further.

HOLD THE COMMENTS

If you see that a friend has lost weight (and even if you think they look great) hold your tongue and consider a more tactful comment you can make instead. For all you know they may have lost weight because they are sick, stressed, depressed or suffering from an eating disorder. You never know if the weight loss has been done in a healthy way. Resist the temptation to comment on someone else's weight (loss or gain) or what they are eating. Rather than commenting on their appearance, simply ask them how they are.

Ashley

Perhaps you can relate to Ashley, whose mother is always commenting on her weight:

'I went to my parents' house for dinner. I went to take more food as I was pretty hungry and then my mum told me off. I couldn't believe it. She made me feel so ashamed. I left, upset, and on my way home I stopped at the shops, bought a bag of chocolate and ate the whole bag. I had been doing so well and was feeling so good about myself and then just the way mum made me feel, I went for chocolate to feel better. I felt worthless and unsuccessful after one incident. I act out, bingeing after every time she makes negative comments about the way I look. My mum has always been very conscious of her weight and I have heard about it as long as I can remember.'

Ashley's mum was trying to help by making a comment about Ashley's weight and food, rationalising, 'If I don't tell her, then who will?' Unfortunately, hearing these judgmental comments about her body and food choices had the opposite effect for Ashley.

Like Claire asking her husband for help, I had enlisted my parents to help me stick to my weight-loss goals. I asked them to hide the lollies so I couldn't find them. By making my parents my 'food police', I put pressure on myself to eat perfectly in front of them. So I would order the healthiest option on the menu and say no to dessert. But when I was alone, I'd find the packet of hidden lollies, sneak spoonfuls of peanut butter and replace missing blocks of chocolate that I had eaten because I felt deprived.

For some people, comments about their weight or food can be triggering in another way. Comments such as 'you've lost weight', 'you look thin' or 'you've gained weight' can lead to restriction and obsession.

If you have a food police or body bully in your life, you need to address it with them. It's scary, it'll be hard (I know!) but it's essential. Once you have communicated your needs, you'll reclaim some control over your body, your eating and behaviour. Many times, the person making the comments or judgements has struggled with their weight, food or body image. They are self-conscious about how they look or overly critical of other people's bodies. When they make comments to you, they are reflecting their insecurities about their own body and their relationship with food. And it's not OK.

To truly heal your relationship with food, to regain control over eating and learn to love your body, you need to communicate with your food police and body bullies. Here are some conversation starters:

- 'I know you're trying to help me, but when you comment on my eating, it makes me want to eat more, not less. It doesn't motivate me to be healthier. In fact, it makes me feel bad about myself.'
- 'I'd love you to support me by not commenting on my weight or what I eat anymore.'

THE PROBLEM IS NOT WITH YOUR BODY. IT'S WITH THE IDEA THAT YOUR BODY MUST LOOK *perfect* IN ORDER TO BE HEALTHY

- 'Even though I've asked for your help before, I found it didn't help the way I thought it would.'
- 'I feel judged when you say xxxxxx and, unfortunately, it doesn't support me to be healthier. I really am trying to be healthier so I'll be trying something different. It's not a fad diet so it will take time. So I need your support.'
- 'If you'd like me to be my happiest and live at my healthiest weight, then please don't comment on my weight, body or what I eat.'

After time, they may forget about the conversation and slip back into old habits. If they require reminders about your wishes, it's really important that you remind them that judgmental comments about your weight, food or body are not OK any more. Try these comments:

- 'I know you're trying to help, by commenting on xxxxx. But I have asked you before not to make these comments. Each time you make these comments, you drive me to xxxxxx and it doesn't help.'
- 'I have asked you really nicely not to comment on my weight/food/body. It's really important that your respect my decision.'

You may need to have this conversation several times before they finally stop trying to police your food intake.

Dealing with sceptics of non-dieting

Non-dieting is very different from the usual restriction, control and deprivation method promoted in the media. This means that your loved ones may be quite sceptical of it. If they don't see how reducing control can actually put you back into the driver's seat, rest assured that it does. There will be sceptics along the way who believe you should get back onto a diet and weigh yourself, but they're still a product of dieting culture. When this happens, politely explain that dieting doesn't work, that there has never been one study to show that diets are effective in the long term and that you're working on being healthy instead. You can also encourage them to read this book.

The definition of insanity is doing the same thing and expecting a different outcome. If you want something you've never had, you need to do something you've never done.

The perfect body *vs* the healthy body

The current 'perfect body' ideal for both men and women is skewed, and it's not healthy, balanced or realistic for most people, even those with the genes to match. Very few people can have the perfect body and a healthy body. You need to redefine what healthy looks like. It's not one shape, it's not abs or the absence of love handles. You can have a soft tummy and still be strong and be healthy. The problem is not with your body. It's with the idea that your body must look 'perfect' in order to be healthy.

It's socially acceptable to be a perfectionist. In fact, we act as though it's an asset: when asked in a job interview about your biggest weakness, you respond with 'perfectionism', intending your 'weakness' to be seen as a strength. Yet perfectionism is not a badge of honour; in fact, being a perfectionist really isn't a strength. It holds you back out of fear that 'I am not good enough' or what you do, create, suggest, deliver is not good enough. This very real, very powerful fear causes perfectionists to:

- Be chronic procrastinators and put things off, sometimes missing deadlines or not delivering the best work you can.
- Say no to or miss out on big opportunities out of fear that you won't meet your own high (unrealistic) expectations. Why bother trying when I know I won't get it perfect?
- Let other people walk over you and undercharge for your time and skills because you don't value your own worth.
- Consistently doubt yourself so simple tasks like writing a paragraph take hours, instead of minutes.

Perfectionism tells you:

- 'You need me. You'd be nothing without me.'
- 'I'm the reason you're successful.'
- 'You always screw up. You never get anything right.'
- 'Next time will be different. I won't hurt you again.'

Because of the things your internal perfectionist tells you, you're too scared to break it off. So you stay stuck in a relationship and mindset that holds you back from being your happiest self.

As long as you are in a relationship with perfectionism, you will never get the love and acceptance of yourself that you so truly deserve. You can never chase and catch perfection. It does not exist. As long as you hold yourself to unattainable standards, expecting perfection from yourself, you'll continue to disappoint yourself.

Do you see yourself properly?

Have you ever (wholeheartedly) loved your body? Think back to what your body has been like, through the years. You've probably been different weights, had a different body shape. At your slimmest weight, do you remember ever feeling 100 per cent delighted with everything about your body? Has there ever been a time when you fully embraced your weight, your size, your shape?

Even at my slimmest, I could always think of something I wanted to change. 'Losing a bit more weight would be nice.' 'My arms are still a bit big.' 'I don't have abs.' 'My bum is too flat.' 'My thighs are still too chunky.' Yet looking back at photos of myself, I think I looked wonderful; of course, I didn't feel incredible at the time. No matter how good my body was, it was never good enough for me (and my unattainable standards).

It's not worth sacrificing your mental health to have the perfect body.

Self-compassion

Self compassion is being able to be compassionate to yourself in moments when you think you've failed, when you feel inadequate or not good enough. Learning self-compassion is one of the most effective ways to push back against perfectionism, increase self-esteem and feel good about yourself.

It's about changing the way you speak to yourself and embracing your perceived flaws.

Self-acceptance

Do you accept yourself for who you are? Accepting yourself is scary. My biggest concern was always this: 'if I accept myself now, as I really am, imperfect and "not there yet", does that mean I'll stop improving?' When people told me to accept my body, I thought that meant I'd never lose weight or be healthy. I thought you had to be thin to be healthy, so if I stopped trying to be thin, then I'd never really get there.

boost your body image

Perfectionism says:

I must be more beautiful and
feminine and popular.
I must never forget things.
My house must always be neat and tidy.
I must be good at everything,
the first time I do it.
She is so much more beautiful than me.
I'm not doing enough;
I should do better

Self-compassion says:

I am perfect the way I am.
It's OK to make mistakes.
The house can be messy; it doesn't
make me less capable.
It's OK not to be good at everything,
especially the first time.
She can be beautiful; it doesn't
make me less beautiful.
I'm doing my best.

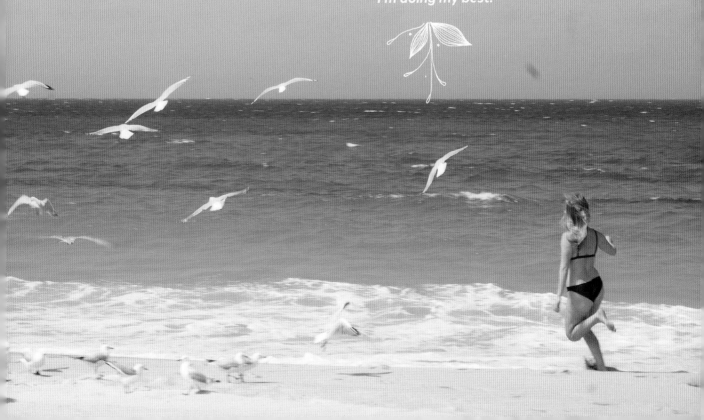

YOU CAN CHOOSE TO ACCEPT YOURSELF AS YOU ARE, *right now*

For years I thought that judging myself would motivate me to be better, but actually it's quite the opposite. When you don't accept yourself as you are, you don't have faith in your own abilities. You second-guess your capacity; you 'um' and 'ah' about doing what you really want; you let other people walk all over you; you find it hard to set healthy boundaries.

Judgments don't lift you up, they tear you down. They keep you stuck in the same old patterns, repeating the same old mistakes. Judgment weighs you down and makes you feel heavier, whereas acceptance makes you feel lighter and brighter.

You won't suddenly become worthy when you lose weight or do a difficult pose in yoga or get that promotion, because the goal posts will just keep moving and you'll forever be chasing acceptance. Soon the voice in your head will pipe up: 'but you could still lose a little more', 'you're not as good as her' or 'soon they're going to realise that I'm not good enough for this role'.

How many years have you been hating your body and feeling unhappy with your weight? Yet you are never truly satisfied. At some point you need to decide that you don't want to keep chasing a goal that doesn't exist. It doesn't matter how long you've been at war with your body, you just need to make the choice to do things differently.

Self-acceptance is a choice. You can choose to accept yourself as you are, right now. No need to get a summer body or be cellulite free. You're imperfect (and that's perfectly OK).

Forgive yourself

Aren't you sick and tried of giving yourself a hard time, all the time? It's empowering to know that you have the ability to decide you're OK, you're enough, you're worthy as you are right now. If you can't muster self-love just yet (baby steps!) then start simply with self-acceptance. Start by muting the voice in your head that says, 'you're not good enough' by deciding that you truly are OK.

The most practical way to begin self-acceptance is to forgive yourself. When you mess up, it's easy to roll through the scenario in your mind, playing out how you could have done better, said something smarter or kept your cool. Forgiving yourself means deciding that you did your best and your best was good enough. It's a relief when you do forgive yourself. I have a mantra I use when I find myself in these situations. It's simply: 'I accept myself and I accept others' or 'I forgive myself'. As soon as you forgive yourself, you can stop mulling over what happened and begin to move on. Your energy can shift again and you become open to a lighter, happier mood. The quicker you can forgive yourself, the sooner the relief will come. Practise this daily and you'll get better at it.

boost your body image

Boost your body image

Body love isn't about losing weight and exercising until you finally love your body. Body love is accepting that your body is imperfect and deciding to love it anyway.

Step 1. Accept that feeling fat has nothing to do with your weight

Changing your weight will not improve your body image. Having poor body image is in your mind. The people with the best bodies in the world often have the worst body image. On the opposite side of the spectrum, there are plenty of people of all shapes who feel really comfortable in their body. In fact, they love their bodies! Looking good in a bikini won't give you better body image. If you want to have better body image, you need to work on your relationship with your body.

Step 2. Swap the 'highlights reel' for real life

Social media is overrun with lean fitness models who have really poor body image. They share selfies of their abs, shot with the perfect lighting, a filter and at the ideal time of day. Then they caption the photo with something about 'balance' or why you need to love your body, yet they continue to sell restrictive diets and intensive exercise plans. You live in a world that doesn't want you to be happy with your body. Being OK with yourself doesn't make money for the beauty, health and fashion industries. You're up against that and it's not easy, but knowing this can help you be kinder to yourself, to forgive yourself when you do notice that you're being harsh on your body.

Case study

Anna

Hating my body and dieting is something I have battled with my whole life. I've tried everything: nothing worked and I felt terrible about myself, a failure. I started reading your blog and loved everything you talked about. I realised I've been hating my body for 20 years, never feeling truly happy. I decided that I've wasted enough time in anguish over my weight and I don't want to spend the rest of my life hating my body. You made me realise that it's up to me to decide that my body is OK; no-one else can give me that.

I decided to stop trying to lose weight and, instead, work on loving my body and being healthy.

My miserable self-image, my constant battle against food and my body, is all changing. It's not easy: it's a work in progress, but I no longer feel that I am unworthy. I feel in control and happy to be myself.

Step 3. Do a social media detox (it's the only detox I recommend!)

Unsubscribe from social media accounts that set unrealistic expectations about what you 'should' look like, or how much you 'should' be exercising or eating. If you feel worse about your body after seeing their snaps, unsubscribe or unfollow. Likewise, if you have any 'friends' who make you feel not pretty, thin or good enough, turn off their notifications so you don't get triggered.

Body love touch

My stomach has been a trouble zone for me and a body part I don't feel so comfortable about. Where others (read: celebrities and models) have abs, I have softness and rolls when I sit down. I have stretchmarks and love handles.

When I feel worried about this part of my body, I find this simple exercise helpful. Run your hands over your body, especially those body parts that you are the most conscious of. For me, I started simply by touching my stomach. Touch your stomach gently and softly, with love and care. Don't grab at your skin, at your fat or your folds (as you normally do). Rather, play with your skin softly, rub it gently and with love. Run your hands over your skin. Focus your attention on the spots that you don't like about your body—your 'trouble' spots.

I'm not going to lie; the first time I did this exercise I felt strange and uncomfortable. It felt so foreign. I realised that I always touch my body in a severe way. This exercise challenged my comfort zone and left me thinking about it for days after.

If touching your own body softly, gently and with love also feels foreign to you, then there even more reason to continue to do this exercise. Did you notice how different that feels, to touch your own body with love instead of discontent and resentment? If someone loves you (a lover, or a parent or child, for example), they touch your body with care and with love. A lover would never grab at your body in such a rough way. If you want to love your body, you also need to change how you touch your body. You must treat and touch your body with respect.

This is a good exercise when you're feeling vulnerable and critical of your body. You may also want to tell yourself: 'I love my body. I love my softness. I love my curves. I love my body unconditionally.' Find the words that resonate with you.

These are the type of words a lover might say to you. These are words of unconditional love. And while you may not feel the meaning in the beginning, sometimes, you need to do the behaviour and the belief will follow.

Loving your body takes practice and patience. You can't wake up one day and suddenly expect to love your body (and know how to love it). You have to work at it. You have to change your language around your body, around the food you nourish it with. You have to consciously change your thinking, challenge those around you and decide to no longer hate your body. Loving your body is a decision and process. Be patient. It's worth it.

Tip

Body love isn't about losing weight and exercising until you finally love your body. Body love is accepting that your body is imperfect and deciding to love it anyway.

Tackle negative self talk

How you talk to yourself matters. Lao Tzu famously said, 'Your thoughts create your world'. The words in your head define who you are and your behaviour. Your mindset matters more than your behaviour because your thoughts are what keep good behaviours going. If you're to make positive changes, and keep up with them, you need to tackle the negative self talk that keeps you stuck, makes you restless at night and prevents you from being exactly who you want to be.

You control your thoughts. Your thoughts control your world.

You may have noticed, there are many voices inside your head that impact how you feel. These voices are very powerful and have the ability to lift you up or break you down or keep you stuck obsessing over the same problems for hours.

There are some key voices you need to be aware of. Perhaps you can relate?

The controller: 'You shouldn't have eaten that. It was too fatty.'

The mean girl: 'You're not good enough. You're not thin enough. You need to lose more weight.'

The rebel: 'Well, you've eaten it already, you may as well finish it.'

The friend: 'You're perfect the way you are. You're hungry so it's time to eat. You've got this.'

Note the voice: once you have awareness, you have the opportunity to adjust your behaviour. So the first step is simply becoming aware of the voice in your head. This is called 'noting'. Note the voice without judgment, just curiosity: 'Oh, I'm giving myself a hard time right now.'

As long as the voice runs free in your brain, it'll keep you stuck feeling sad, controlled, angry or ashamed. Once you've noted the voice with curiosity, it's time to forgive and accept yourself. By processing the emotion instead of trying to control or ignore, you're able to move through it. Once I started doing this, I found I could come out of a bad mood much quicker.

When the controller says, 'You shouldn't have eaten that. It was too fatty,' you reply, 'I was hungry. It's exactly what I felt like.'

When the mean girl says, 'You're not good enough. You're not thin enough. You need to lose more weight,' you respond with, 'I accept my body as it is. I am doing my best. I am exactly where I need to be.'

If the rebel negotiates: 'Well, you've eaten it already, you may as well finish it,' you tell yourself, 'I trust my body to guide me.'

You are capable of doing difficult things, things that scare you and challenge you. Like asking for help. Or saying no. Or walking down the beach wearing a bikini. Or trying even though you think you'll fail. You are stronger than you think.

Affirmations

I used to think affirmations were silly, trivial and didn't do much. Then I started doing them. Most affirmations I had read before didn't resonate with me, so I made up my own. At first I started small: you are OK as you are; I accept myself and I accept others; you screwed up but it's still OK. Then, I progressed and my affirmations became clearer and stronger.

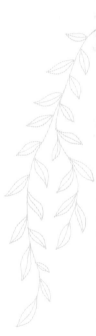

You deserve to be happy.
You are enough.
You are worthy of love.
You are freaking awesome.
You are stronger than you realise.
You've got this.

Often, you need to do things before you feel you're ready. Like giving up smoking before you want to or saying affirmations before you believe they are true. Do the behaviour and your brain will change with you.

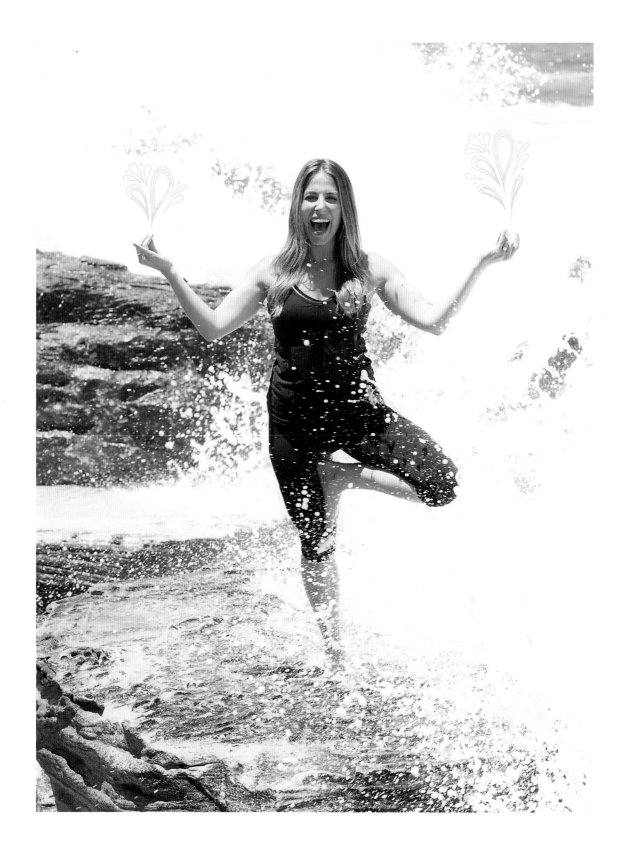

7

feel amazing

For me, one of the best indicators of your health is the way you feel. Healthy is when you have the energy to do the things you love. Food has a big role to play in this, but so does exercise, sleep, stress, alcohol and drugs. Considering the whole body—and all of the things that influence your health—can help you balance your hormones, mood and energy.

When your hormones and mood are balanced and you've got plenty of energy, you feel amazing. Food plays an important role in balancing your hormones, mood and energy, but there are a number of other factors to consider.

Do you feel low on energy, as though you're just getting through the day? Struggle with mood swings? Your hormones are your body's chemical messengers. They move around your body, delivering messages between different cells and organs. Hormones work hard to make sure important things get done.

When your hormones are off balance (too high or too low) or overworked, it can really impact on your mood, skin, periods, sleep quality, energy levels, weight, libido and appetite. By making a few simple lifestyle tweaks, you can start to feel like your best version of yourself.

There are a few things you can do to help rebalance your hormones naturally, but your first stop should be to see your doctor who can refer you to an endocrinologist if necessary. Otherwise, try the following things to give your body the best chance of hormonal balance:

1. Eat enough healthy fats.
Your body can't make hormones when it doesn't have the right building blocks. Many hormones are fat-soluble, so getting enough 'healthy' fats, and a good variety, in your diet will help prevent hormonal imbalances. Good sources include avocado, extra virgin olive oil, avocado oil, macadamia oil, walnuts, chia seeds and linseeds (flaxseeds).

2. Prioritise quality sleep.
It doesn't matter how 'healthy' the rest of your life is, if you don't get enough sleep, your

IMBALANCE IN HORMONES MAY BE CAUSED BY:

- A lack of quality sleep or rest (including shift work)
- High stress levels and demanding work hours
- Drinking alcohol
- Unhealthy balance of gut bacteria
- Eating too much processed, sugary food
- Exposure to chemicals
- Overexercising
- Genetics

cortisol levels increase, which can slow your metabolism, increase hunger and mess with your energy and mood. Make sleep a priority. See my tips on page 136 to help you improve your sleeping patterns.

3. Sidestep the chemicals.
Pesticides, pollution, cosmetics, household cleaning products and plastics may contain xeno-oestrogens that can mimic hormones in the body, upsetting the balance of your hormones. Reducing the amount of chemicals in your life can help restore oestrogen levels. Wash fruit and vegetables well, buy organic if

you can afford it, use nonplastic water bottles, eat foods containing phyto-oestrogens, avoid heating foods in plastic containers or use BPA-free[1] plastics, skip parabens in cosmetics and choose low-chemical cleaning products or make your own: lemon, vinegar and bicarbonate of soda (baking soda) are great!

4. Consume foods with phyto-oestrogens.
Phyto-oestrogens are a natural compound found in some vegetables, fruit, seeds, nuts, healthy oils, wholegrains and some herbs. They can help prevent your body from absorbing harmful xeno-oestrogens. Add these foods into your diet: beetroot (beets), cabbage, carrots, corn, beans, garlic, parsley, peas, lentils, kidney beans, potatoes, pumpkin (squash), soy products, split peas, squash, yams, zucchini (courgettes); apples, cherries, plums, pomegranate, rhubarb; gluten-containing wholegrains such as barley, oats, rye, wheat (and wheatgerm); and 'healthy' fats such as linseeds (flaxseeds), extra virgin olive oil, peanut oil and safflower oil.

5. Exercise.
When it comes to exercise, more is not always better. Overexercising can lead to burnout and imbalances for your thyroid and adrenal glands. Find exercise you enjoy, be sure to take enough rest days to recover and develop a healthy relationship with exercise. See my tips starting on page 126.

6. Add probiotics.
Many important neurotransmitters are created in the gut so maintaining a healthy balance of gut bacteria is essential. Eating foods that contain probiotics is a fantastic way to boost the 'good' bacteria in your gut. Greek-style yoghurt is a great source of probiotics, so a serve a day is a good idea. Why not try Get-up-and-go oats on page 155 or adding Cheeky tzatziki (see page 210) as a condiment to meals. Enjoy fermented foods like kimchi, sauerkraut, kombucha and kefir, if you like.

7. Boost fibre intake.
Fibrous foods often contain prebiotics (which are food for probiotics). Eat plenty of vegetables with the skin on, snack on fresh fruit, add seeds and nuts to salads and enjoy beans at least three times a week.

8. Eat more wholefoods.
Eating too much processed, sugary food can unbalance your insulin levels, causing big highs and lows in energy and mood and increasing fat storage around your belly. If you're having banana bread for breakfast, drinking soft drink (soda), having biscuits (cookies) with tea and coffee and relying on lollies (candy or sweets) to get you through the 3 pm slump every day, your insulin levels may be out of balance. Using the balanced meal guide (on pages 72–73) and eating more wholefoods will help you feel more energised and may reduce your risk of diseases like diabetes.

9. Manage stress.

Feel like you have a never-ending to-do list? High levels of stress can bump up cortisol (your stress hormone). Spikes in cortisol levels can make you hungry and create cravings for high-carbohydrate and sugary foods (that's why it's called stress eating)! Stress is a normal and inevitable part of life, but when you have too much stress or don't have healthy coping mechanisms, your hormones and neurotransmitters can become imbalanced. If you're feeling stressed regularly, you may need to make some lifestyle changes to reduce your stress and adopt strategies to help you cope better with stress. If necessary, speak with a psychologist or counsellor.

10. Cut back on booze.

Alcohol can throw off your hormones, particularly if you're drinking a lot. Alcohol impacts on the quality of your sleep, which is crucial for healthy hormones. Binge-drinking on the weekends is particularly tough on your body and can bump up your weight. When it comes to alcohol, less is best.

Balancing your mood

If you always feel stressed, tired, anxious or overwhelmed, it doesn't matter how well you're doing or healthily you're eating, you won't feel good. It's so important to invest in your mood and energy levels. I've always struggled with mood swings and anxiety but with some work and strategies, I've learned how to keep my mood more stable and I feel so much better for it.

My struggle with anxiety

Looking back, I can see that I was always anxious. But when I was finally diagnosed with clinical anxiety 10 years ago, I was in shock. At the same time, I was also so relieved to be diagnosed, because it helped me adopt strategies that make me feel so much better. Even if you don't have a known mental-health condition like anxiety or depression, many of the things I've learned by managing my anxiety will also help you deal with stress, overwhelming feelings and exhaustion.

The power of routine, rituals and habits

It's hard to have room for joy and happiness and time to be playful when things feel out of order and overwhelming. Strong routines and habits can help you get the foundations right so you feel grounded. From there, you can add layers into your life that make it feel really, really good.

But being too rigid with rituals can also be a problem. As with all things, there's got to be balance. If you're too rigid with routines and can't embrace spontaneity, then you need to embrace ambiguity. This may mean going out to dinner with your friends instead going to the gym every so often, just to remind yourself that routines aren't rules. There's always a choice.

I'm not naturally a fan of routines. I'm not a morning person. And I prefer spontaneity over schedules. For years, I resisted daily rituals because they sounded boring and I was scared that they would lock me down, stifle my creativity and prevent me from ever doing anything exciting. But I was wrong.

Setting up healthy routines, rituals and habits helps you get through your to-do list, which decreases stress and anxiety. You achieve more in the day, leaving room for the good stuff. Thanks to supportive routines like exercise and sleep schedules, healthy habits are less likely to fall through and you feel better, stronger and healthier. I've certainly found that embracing healthy rituals can help you live healthier and happier, with less anxiety and more balance.

Your hormones

Cortisol – Stress hormone.
Cortisol is released when you feel stressed. It impacts your blood-sugar levels, immune system and blood pressure and can cause fat to be stored around your belly.

Adrenaline – Fight-or-flight hormone.
The quickening heartbeat when you get nervous is caused by adrenaline. Adrenaline is also released when you feel stressed.

Insulin – Fat-storing hormone.
Insulin is released to help your body process the carbohydrates in food. Highly processed junk food tends to cause a big spike in insulin levels because of the high sugar content. Insulin affects how your body stores fat, making it harder to lose weight.

Serotonin – Happy hormone.
When you eat delicious food serotonin is released, making you feel good. Serotonin is also important for good sleep and appetite.

Oestrogen – Fertility hormone.
Healthy oestrogen levels are important for fertility and reproduction. Oestrogen imbalance can be caused by exposure to xeno-oestrogens, which are man-made chemicals often found in plastics, cosmetics, pesticides and cleaning products. It is thought that chronically high levels of oestrogen can make you more likely to be insulin resistant.

Leptin – Fullness hormone.
Leptin is the satiety hormone that is released in your body after a meal to let you know that you've had enough food. It's an essential hormone for hunger and metabolism.

Ghrelin – Hunger hormone.
When you feel hunger, it's because ghrelin has been released into your body, reminding you that it's time to refuel. When you're stressed and don't get enough sleep, your body releases more ghrelin, so you get more energy from food when you can't sleep.

T3 and T4 (thyroid hormone[2]) – Metabolism hormones.
These hormones play an important role in metabolism, mood, weight and energy. An underactive thyroid can make it really difficult to lose weight.

Testosterone – Sex hormone.
Impacts your sex drive and regulates how you build muscle.

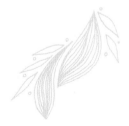

Healthy routine basics

Wake up at the same time every day.
This will help your body clock get into a stable, healthy routine, help balance your hormones and mood and make it easier for you to wake up. Go to bed at the same time each night. This'll make getting enough sleep each night much more doable. Make sleep a priority.

Plan your exercise for the week.
Book in classes, make plans with friends or simply write down the days you plan to exercise and put it in your diary. Sometimes gentle exercise every morning is easier to do than vigorous exercise three times a week because you're in a predictable daily routine.

Have set nights when you cook.
Monday, Tuesday and Wednesday tend to be less busy. Scheduling in time to cook these nights will help you cook at home more often. Try some of the dinner recipes in this book.

Keep a calendar.
Schedule routine into your life and it's far more likely to happen. Schedule in a healthy grocery shopping trip on the weekend and meal prep time on Sunday.

Make it practical.
Does your routine actually fit in to your everyday life? The best routines are convenient and realistic. Keep it real. Choose a gym close to you. Order your shopping online. Make it easy and realistic.

Action breeds motivation.
Start a simple routine, even if you think you'd like to do more later on. Thanks to Newton, we know that an object in motion stays in motion. Starting small is all you really need to do, then build from there.

I start my day with a coffee, not warm water with lemon. If you love the ritual (truly and deeply) of lemon juice in warm water, then keep doing it, but try to drink it through a reusable straw because drinking lemon juice every day can be really corrosive for your teeth.

Be firm and flexible.
Know when to prioritise sticking to your routine, and when to be spontaneous. You've got to be flexible so you don't miss out on life. Come back to the routine. Anytime you feel out of control, for example after a holiday, return to the healthy routine. It's incredibly grounding.

Schedule in at least two hours a week for you.
This may mean asking someone else to mind the kids so you can reset, or exercising, or spending some time on Sunday doing nothing. Make yourself a priority and schedule in your own time.

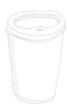

Reality checking

Fill in the boxes. Do this exercise whenever you feel overwhelmed, depressed, stressed or anxious.

When I feel overwhelmed and stuck in my head, I find this simple brain exercise helps me work through my anxiety.

What am I feeling?	What triggered this feeling?	What are my beliefs or assumptions?	What is the reality?	What action can I take?
I feel... overwhelmed; it all feels too hard.	I'm getting so many emails; my to-do list is never-ending.	I don't want to disappoint anyone; I'm scared of offending people.	I don't need to respond to emails immediately; clear boundaries are good for everyone.	Set up an auto-reply to help manage my inbox; ask friends and family for support.
I feel... people are taking advantage of me; underappreciated, annoyed, angry.	People keep asking too much from me; I give and no one gives back.	I feel obligated to help in case people think I am mean; my friends and family don't value my time.	My friends and family do care about me; I need to look after myself first. They will still love me.	Write down the words I need to say next time someone asks me to help; practise saying no; ask people for help.
I feel...				
I feel...				
I feel...				
I feel...				
I feel...				
I feel...				
I feel...				
I feel...				

10 things to help manage your mood

1 Don't wait until you're drowning to put on a life vest

Preventing anxiety, stress or overwhelming emotions from taking over (and engulfing you!) is key. I used to wait until I was drowning in anxiety to do the things that make me feel better; things like enjoyable exercise, saying no, taking a lunch break, meditating, seeing my counsellor and making room for downtime. Now I do these things daily—before I get anxious—and I don't struggle with anxiety as much (or as deeply) as I used to.

2 Exercise for your mental health first, your physical health second

Exercise is the best natural mood booster. Getting a hit of endorphins helped me come off medication and it's one of the ways I treat my anxiety naturally. I exercise, almost daily, to feel good, to have more energy and keep my mood stable. Any additional benefit is just a bonus. Move your body daily, even if it's just gentle exercise, to help balance your mood. Don't underestimate the value of a gentle walk or a 10-minute stretching session.

3 Build (and maintain) a life that boosts your mood

When you feel happy, it's tempting to stop doing the things that help you feel grounded, in control and free from stress. But it's essential to keep the habits consistent. If you are prone to stress, anxiety and being overwhelmed, accept it and then build your life to support and prevent it. Don't stop doing those things that keep you feeling grounded.

4 No-one can read your mind

People don't know what you're feeling if you don't tell them. Don't assume someone (especially your partner) should know you well enough to intuit how you're feeling, and then get upset when they don't automatically 'get it'. Instead of guessing what's on their mind, explain how you're feeling. If you don't tell them when you're struggling or when they've hurt you, they won't know. Have an open conversation. It's scary, I know! But the hard conversations are the most important conversations.

5 Know when anxiety is talking

Is it you or your anxiety talking? Anxiety will often jump to conclusions, make black-and-white statements and blow things out of proportion. For example, anxiety will say things like, 'I've ruined everything', 'They'll never want to work with me again' or 'She didn't call. No one cares about me.' Simply identifying that anxiety (or stress) is speaking can help distance yourself from the feelings. Try the reality check exercise on page 123: do this exercise when you feel overwhelmed, depressed, stressed or anxious.

6 Have a chat

You go to the gym for your physical health but what do you do proactively to look after your mental health? I see a counsellor once a fortnight. Proudly. Speaking to a mental health care professional isn't just for people who are struggling. Seeing a counsellor has made me stronger, more resilient and allowed me to accomplish so much. Now I don't dread going back to work on Monday. There is such relief in having someone who will listen to you, who can be unbiased, but help you recognise patterns and habits you haven't seen before. As professionals, they're impartial and trained to help. Find someone you really like (it's about developing a good relationship). If you don't connect with them, keep looking.

7 Talk about mental health

If you have anxiety or depression, it's OK (no, it's really helpful) to turn to your loved ones (the ones who understand) and share insights into your mental health, such as, 'I'm having an anxious day because...' or 'I'm feeling depressed at the moment...' People often feel awkward talking about mental health, but it's OK not to be OK. And you need to be brave enough to talk about it. Saying the words is the hardest part and it gets easier and easier. If you know someone who has anxiety and depression (or any other mental health condition), ask them how they are feeling. If someone had a broken leg or the 'flu, you'd ask how they are. This is how we need to think of mental health. Simply ask, 'How are you feeling at the moment? Are you OK?'

8 Choose to see your mental condition as strength

In many ways, anxiety has made me stronger. It's made me a lot more empathetic and understanding as a friend. When others are hurting, because I've been there before, I know the pain and I get it. So I'm happy to sit with them, without judgment. Anxiety also allows me to do what I do (help people who struggle with out-of-control eating let go of guilt, restriction, and comparison). I've been there myself, so I'm driven—not by money or fame— but because I want to teach others what I wish I had known when I was struggling, too. What does your stress or anxiety teach you? Does it make you stronger in any way?

9 Eat a healthy diet

You feel good when you eat a healthy diet. Like exercise, eat well because it makes you feel good. Making some simple changes to your diet, as outlined in this book, can help you feel better. Try making the recipes from this book to eat a more Mediterranean-style, mental-health-boosting diet.

10 Consider change, big or small

If you're constantly feeling overwhelmed or stressed and you hate Mondays, then it's a clue that something needs to change. But don't be afraid, it doesn't have to be a big change. Sometimes small changes, such as taking a lunch break, turning off your phone after 7 pm or prioritising self-care and sleep, can make a big difference.

Create a healthy relationship with exercise

I used to exercise to burn calories so I could lose weight. Truly, that was my only reason for going to the gym: will I look good after this? This meant I punished myself with exercise I hated. As a result, exercise was always a chore. I hated it and so I was inconsistent, and this made me feel guilty, unfit and unhealthy. Can you relate?

When you have a healthy relationship with exercise, you enjoy moving your body, which means that you are so much more likely to be consistent. And more than anything, the trick to exercise is consistency. When I stopped punishing myself with gruelling workouts and embraced enjoyable movement, my relationship with exercise improved dramatically. Exercise to feel good, boost your mood, give you energy, keep your gut functioning and your blood circulating, balance your hormones and boost your sex drive.

The power of enjoyable (and gentle) exercise

Like food and eating, you need balance with exercise. This means finding the right mix of exercises to suit you during your specific life stage. I used to think that I had to sweat and be in pain to be exercising properly. 'Feel the burn' was my mantra. But hardcore exercise tore up my body and left me weaker, not stronger.

Even if you aren't sweating or hurting, your body is still benefiting. Don't underestimate the power of gentle exercise. Gentle exercise, such as yoga, walking, swimming and dancing, is incredibly good for you, increases your lifespan and gives you a great dose of endorphins, which boost your mood. Plus, gentle exercise is most often really enjoyable so you're more likely to want to do it. My advice? Swap intensity for consistency.

When I stopped dieting, I also forfeited intensive exercise and I gave myself permission to do slow, enjoyable exercise. Now, exercise

REDISCOVER THE JOY OF GENTLE MOVEMENT

Find exercise that you enjoy, that doesn't feel like punishment. Here are some ideas:

- A walk with your best friend or while listening to a great podcast
- Yoga (and it doesn't have to be Bikram or Vinyasa).
- Stretching
- Dance class
- Swimming
- Tai chi
- A leisurely bike ride through a park

truly is something I look forward to. I never groan when I see it in my diary. In my current exercise routine, I include both gentle and intense exercise. I love going for walks and yoga, and but I also still love beach runs, Pilates, swimming and high-intensity interval training (HIIT). These days, I actually really enjoy some high-intensity exercise. It can burn and feel tough but also feels good and right.

Exercise is your reward, not your punishment

So often I hear people say, 'I have to go the gym tomorrow' after finishing a big meal. That's not balance, that's punishment for eating. Don't exercise because you feel guilty for eating. Exercise because you can. Exercise because it feels good. Exercise because you have the right, the freedom, the money, the time, the opportunity. Don't exercise because you ate too much.

feel amazing

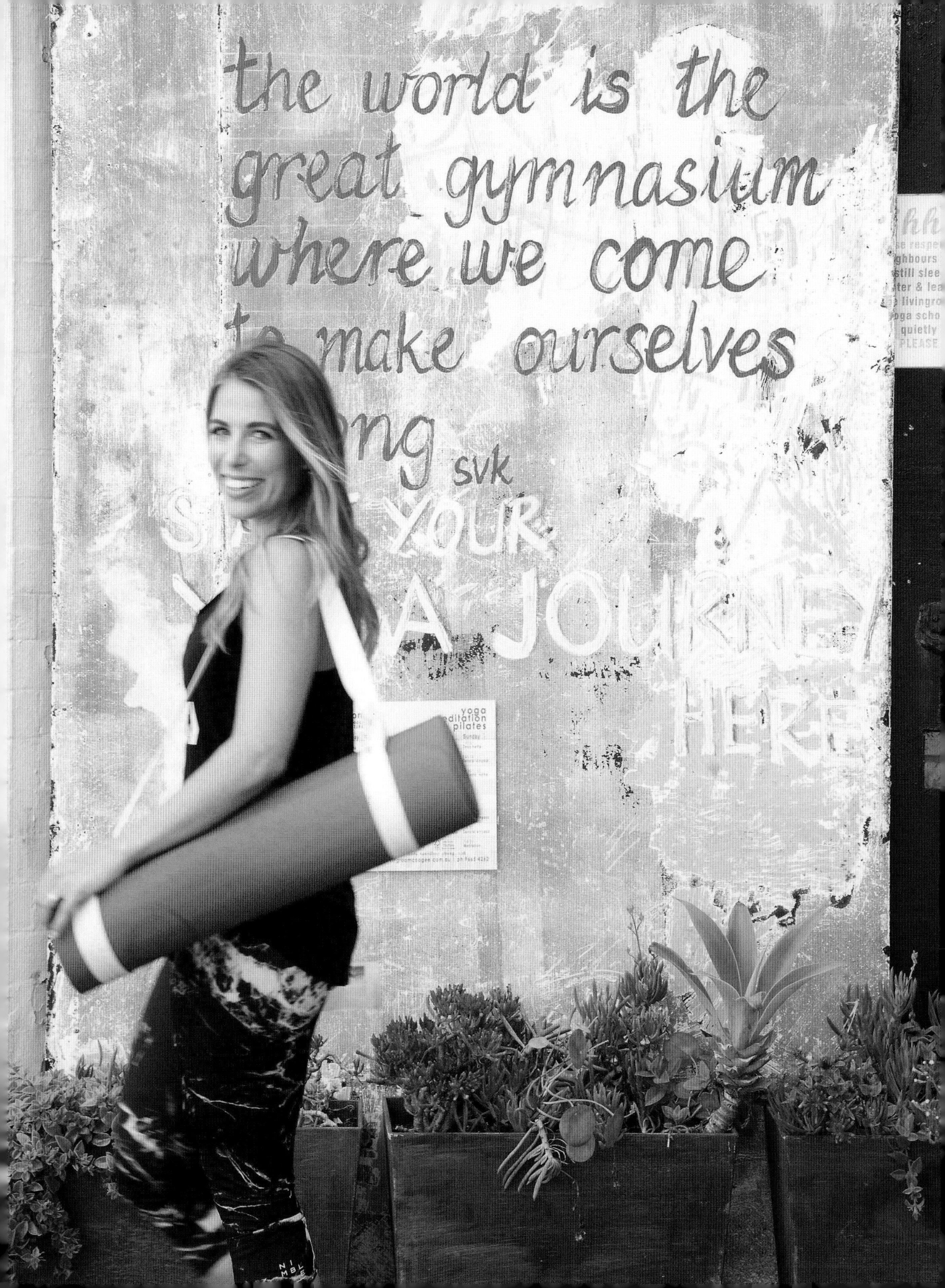

the world is the
great gymnasium
where we come
to make ourselves

...ng svk

...YOUR

...A JOURNEY

HERE

yoga
meditation
pilates

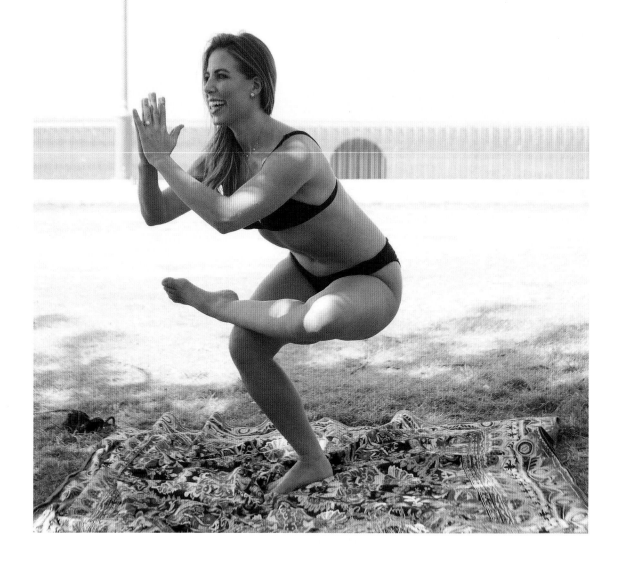

I bend so
I don't break

It really helps to see exercise as a reward. Instead of telling yourself, 'I have to exercise today', remind yourself, 'I am lucky to be able to exercise today'. If I get through a big chunk of work, I reward myself with a walk. I exercise as a thank you to my body and because it feels good. I'm grateful for that luxury.

Overexercising

Overexercising is worse than not exercising at all. When you overexercise you're hurting your body, messing with your hormones and you get weaker instead of stronger. How do you know when you're overexercising?

- Your muscles, joints or bones are always sore. You're constantly stiff, always struggling to walk downstairs or sit.
- You stop getting your period.
- You're always tired.
- You are inflexible with your workouts. You're unable to see friends or deviate from your schedule.
- You feel guilty or anxious when you miss one workout.
- You feel worse after exercise, not better.
- You resent exercising because it feels like punishment.

You should always feel better after you exercise, not worse. If you feel worse, chances are you're pushing yourself too hard. You need to rest or you need to soften up your exercise to be gentler. Rest is healthy. Punishing yourself with gruelling exercise is not.

Are you able to adjust your exercise plans based on how you're feeling physically and emotionally? Do you feel uncomfortable or 'bad' if you cancel your exercise plans? It's really healthy to be flexible with your exercise plans and goals. Staying rigid and set on how much you have to exercise isn't healthy or balanced. Sometimes, you need to be OK with not exercising. Having goals is great but being flexible within those goals is essential. Your fitness and exercise should support your life and give you energy to do the things you

want to do. For many people, exercise starts to control your life, get in the way of life and stops you from doing the things you want to do.

Ask yourself: Do I enjoy the exercise I do? What would I find more enjoyable? How can i make exercise more pleasurable?

Exercising outdoors

Being out in nature can help you feel good, especially if you live in the city. Whenever I get the chance, I like to exercise outside. Wherever you are, plan some exercise outdoors to help boost serotonin and get a healthy dose of vitamin D from the sunshine.

Case study

Jenny

Exercise always felt like a chore for Jenny. When she was dieting, going for a walk never felt like enough, so she pushed herself through exercise she hated. Soon enough, she would stop exercising altogether, then felt guilty and unfit until she threw herself back into a heavy routine of exercise.

Since embracing gentle exercise, Jenny has started getting up 45 minutes earlier each day to go for a walk. She has found she really enjoys the peaceful early morning and it's a great way to start the day. She feels so relaxed and good about herself. Now Jenny sees things differently and because her mindset has shifted, she is accomplishing exercise, self-care and a healthy sleep routine all at the same time. The best bit? Jenny loves it and exercise no longer feels like a chore. This is all because she stopped doing painful and hard exercise she hated.

Angie

I love exercise; it always makes me feel better! But some weeks I exercise every day and other weeks, I don't exercise at all. I really want to become more consistent with exercise. I've got three young children so I'm currently doing 20–30 minutes on the stationary bike, but I can't say I love it. My goal is to be consistently exercising five times a week. What can you recommend?

This is a great goal, because when it comes to health benefits, consistency is key. Regularly exercising (and enjoying it!) will help balance your mood, give you more energy and keep you grounded. Sounds like you're really busy, but prioritising regular exercise is so beneficial and it can be done.

Start small with realistic goals. Aim to exercise two or three times a week, instead of trying to exercise five times a week from the start. Once you consistently exercise on those days, then you can add another day into the routine until you're exercising five days week. When you start small and build, it's far more realistic and doable.

Find exercise you enjoy. The stationary bike might be convenient, but it doesn't sound like you're passionate or enjoying the process. Write a list of the activities you do find enjoyable. If you need to stay at home, then perhaps a DVD workout with music or an online exercise program will be more fun.

Schedule exercise (and rest days) in your diary. If you block out the time, and tell those around you who need to know (like your partner or baby sitters), you'll be more likely to follow through. Allow enough rest days between to recover.

Exercise at the same time of day. Just like waking up at the same time each morning helps you rise, exercising at the same time can help you form a routine. Sometimes, it's easier to exercise every day for a shorter period of time than to exercise every other day. You may find you're less likely to postpone sessions until tomorrow.

Sign up to structure. Having direction can really help inspire your workouts. Sign up to a body resistance, HIIT program if you want to get fitter faster. You don't need any equipment and can do it from anywhere! If you have more flexibility, sign up to a regular gym class like Zumba, Pilates, yoga or barre.

Call a friend. Exercising with friends is wonderful because you catch up with your pal, get a hit of endorphins and the time flies by quicker. You'll also be far less likely to cancel on your friend. Set up a weekly walk while the kids are at sports training or take the kids to a park and workout together. Make it a standing arrangement each week and exercise will be much more consistent (and fun!)

Download a good podcast or listen to music. Listening while I walk helps me learn, groove or be pulled into a great story while exercising. This multitasking will make the time fly and make exercise something to look forward to.

Making (not finding) time for exercise

It sure can be hard to make time to exercise, but it is possible and I believe you deserve it. For me, I have a few life check points that help me know when I'm feeling like I have enough time and I'm not working too hard.

- Am I getting eight to nine hours of sleep?
- Do I have time to cook dinner?
- Do I have time to exercise?

As soon as I no longer have time for these three things, it's a reminder to myself to pull back and reprioritise myself. Preventing burn-out is so important, because once you fall apart, get sick or exhausted, it's a whole lot harder to dig yourself out.

This isn't another 'to-do' list but rather a self-love list. I won't compromise on these points because I deserve these three simple things. What would be on your list?

Put yourself first

If you're constantly giving, people will continue to take. You need to teach people how to treat you. In order to be kind to yourself, you need to practise putting yourself first and that can sometimes mean saying no. Saying no is short-term discomfort so you don't feel long-term resentment. This is easier said than done, but well worth practising.

Saying 'no' without guilt

When you say no more often, you put yourself first and have more time and space for yourself. Saying 'no' sure is tough. We've been trained to be 'nice', which often means putting the needs of others before our own. But saying 'yes' to every request that comes your way has serious consequences for your physical and mental health.

Learning to put yourself first and say no isn't easy, especially if you've been looking out for everyone else for many years. Practising self-care (without feeling guilty) is one of the biggest gifts you can give to yourself and those you love.

CREATE YOUR OWN SELF-LOVE LIST

If you find you consistently don't have time for yourself or exercise, it might be time to prioritise yourself and start saying no a little more often. What are three things you need to do for yourself every day (or almost every day) to feel aligned and cared for?

1. _____

2. _____

3. _____

Saying 'no' isn't selfish. The truth is you can't be the best friend, partner, daughter, sister, mother, aunty or colleague when you're exhausted and burnt out. When you put others' needs first and neglect your own needs, you'll:

- Resent your loved ones for not helping you more
- Be exhausted, overworked and overtired
- Have lower immunity, so you're more likely to get sick
- Be sapped of your energy
- Not be able to live the happiest, fullest life you deserve

Oprah, the queen of, well, everything, says that you must teach people how to treat you. So how are you teaching people to treat you?

Are you setting boundaries or are others setting boundaries for you?

Are you voicing your opinion or letting others make all the decisions?

Do you make everyone else a delicious healthy lunch for the next day, but don't make one for yourself?

Do you resent those around you for not being more considerate?

Do you feel people are sometimes taking advantage of you or taking you for granted?

Do you feel underappreciated?

If so, it's time to teach them how to treat you. You can't wait for them to realise that it's not ok to keep asking of you without giving back. You must teach them how you deserve and expect to be treated.

Setting healthy boundaries

Setting clear boundaries always scared me. What if they think I'm rude? What if no-one likes me anymore? What if they think I'm selfish, mean, and not committed to the greater good? Chances are some people may think those things. But most people will respect you more for setting clear, and healthy boundaries. They will see you thrive, regain energy and become a happier person. Everyone wins. Setting clear and healthy boundaries will help you show up in the world you want, instead of feeling like you're everyone else's slave.

You can't sacrifice yourself so others will be happy. It's your responsibility to take care of yourself first. No one else is going to do it. People will be very comfortable asking you for favours, especially if you're always saying yes. Soon enough, those favours become expectations and your list of 'things to do' continues to grow until it's overwhelming and feels incredibly unfair (and unsustainable).

Like all things, practice makes it easier to say no. Having the right words, and practising saying them, can help make saying no easier. Here are some lines I find useful:

- Thanks for asking but I'm really busy and prioritising my time.
- I'd love to help but I can't.

- I don't have the time and need to really focus on me/my family/my work.
- I'm not able to help right now, but why not ask ... for help

Say 'no' now so you don't resent it later. Saying no isn't as scary as you think. Each time you practise saying it, it gets easier. Chances are, you overestimate how much saying 'no' will effect the person asking. Take note of how the person responds. Do they scream at you and get angry? Or do they simply say, 'OK' and move on to ask someone else?

Guilt will make you doubt your decision. As soon as you say no, guilt may creep into you head and you may contemplate taking it back, but stand your ground. Push through the discomfort, the guilt and the desire to jump in and do it all yourself. You need to stand by your decision, even in the discomfort of guilt.

When to say yes

- When the idea excites you
- When you won't resent it later
- When you benefit deeply from the activity
- When you have enough time

Give for yourself.

Saying no is hard, but it's still easier than regretting that you said yes.

feel amazing ◠◠◠

RUSHING AROUND ISN'T GOOD FOR YOUR *health* OR RELATIONSHIPS

Self-care

You can't pour from an empty cup. Self-care isn't a luxury, it's a necessity and missing out on self-care can set you up for burn-out, anxiety and depression, smoking, numbing behaviours such as drinking alcohol, taking drugs and binge eating, unhealthy eating habits and stress.

Self-care doesn't have to be 'hippy-dippy' or feel like just one more thing on your to-do list. It's important to work out what self-care feels like for you. It's different for all of us. Self-care for you might be going for a bushwalk one week or having a nap the next. Create a self-care habit. Self-care isn't something you do once or twice and then forget about. It's a ritual and habit to bring into your life. The best self-care practice is when you choose practical ideas. Getting a weekly massage sounds amazing but fitting this into the schedule and budget may cause more stress than it relieves.

Sometimes self-care is getting up early to exercise. Other times, self-care is sleeping in. Here are some self-care ideas:

- Have a nap
- Take a bath
- Bake or cook something fun
- Do a craft project, paint or sew
- Create a compliments file where you store the nice things people have said about you. It's easy to forget these things and jump to big conclusions when you're feeling exhausted, anxious or stressed.
- Play a sport or join a dance class
- Exercise for an endorphin hit
- Go on a bushwalk or take your pet for a walk
- If you're overly tired or getting sick, not exercising can be also be self-care
- Call a close friend
- Do something that will make you happy, instead of doing what other people want
- Don't check social media or emails for a day or weekend
- Have a manicure or pedicure
- Visit the library or a museum and get lost for a few hours
- Turn off your phone
- Stretch
- Read a book
- See a counsellor or psychologist

Personally, I prefer to practise self-care every day by taking a lunch break, exercising and reading for an hour before bed. This prevents me burning out and helps me enjoy the working week more.

Embrace un-busy-ness

I'm guilty of always being in a rush, but those who live in areas of the world where the people live long and happy lives embrace a slower way of life. Rushing around isn't good for your health or your relationships. Here are a few tips for slowing down:

- Allow plenty of time to avoid getting frustrated in traffic.
- Set a schedule that suits you. You don't have to bend to other people's schedules. Sometimes they can meet when it suits you.
- Un-busy yourself. Once a month, plan a weekend where you have no commitments.
- Say 'yes' to things that make you feel excited, but say 'no' when your gut says, 'Are you sure you've got time'?

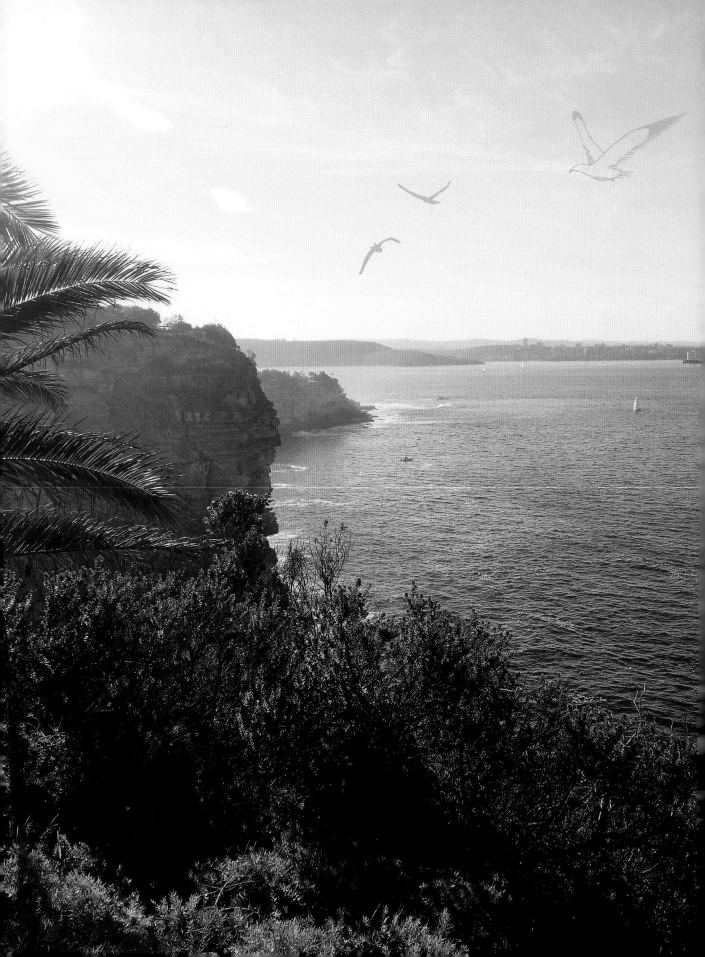

Connections and relationships

There is so much more to life than social media makes out. I truly believe the only things that matter in life are relationships and health. Meaningful relationships create a sense of belonging: community and connection help you live a longer, healthier and happier life.

Got a friend whose excessive drinking, gossiping, smoking or relationship with food makes it hard for you to live healthily? Don't underestimate how much the people around you influence your wellbeing. You have options: try seeing them for breakfast walks instead of after-work cocktails. Help encourage them to make changes (ones that, of course, have nothing to do with weight). Or have the hard conversation so that your friendship can grow stronger in a more supportive way.

Having trouble with an important relationship? Please consider speaking to a psychologist or counsellor.

Healthy technology use

Mobile phones and devices are part of our lives. My phone has been the cause of a lot of my anxiety and I wasn't even aware. While technology can cause anxiety, it can also be incredibly helpful, so I don't believe in boycotting it: instead, I prefer to embrace technology, but on my terms. By creating healthy technology habits, I feel so much better about my body, my life and myself. Here are some essential strategies I depend on to have a healthy relationship with technology.

1. Turn off buzzing and sound notifications on your phone.

When you check your phone, even if you don't respond, you are sending a message to the person you're speaking to that your phone is more important than them. You'll have much stronger, healthier relationships with this simple change.

Tip

Keep unfollowing people in your newsfeed every few months (like getting rid of unwanted clothes in our wardrobe) to keep your newsfeed healthy and balanced.

2. Close your email tabs or program for at least two hours each day.

Emails are a constant distraction that demand your attention NOW! But you don't need to respond to email immediately (people can call you if it's truly urgent). When I want to be productive (like right now as I am writing this book), I close my email or turn off my wifi.

3. Social media detox.

See page 113 for some tips.

4. Beware of scrolling.

Scroll with intent, not aimlessly. Pinterest can be helpful for inspiration, but it can also make you feel like your life isn't glamorous enough. On Instagram, be weary of the 'explore' feed, which is filled with images of perfect-looking models or girls in crop tops with abs, drinking green juices. These images are not real life and can be incredibly tough on your self-esteem.

5. Track your usage.

How many hours a day do you think you use your phone? Scrolling can be a massive time suck. Be clear on how long you want to spend on social media each time. Download an app that will track how much you use your phone. It'll also tell you which apps you use the most. Be warned: the results may alarm you!

6. Embrace white space.

I'm not talking about home decor. Like most of us, you are probably so busy, that any time you have a moment free from 'doing' something, you are tempted to fill that white space by checking your phone, emails, or social media. Constantly filling this white space can add to the feeling of busyness and make you feel overwhelmed and overstretched. It's incredibly tempting to fill that time waiting (for a friend to arrive at a café, for a bus, for the food to cook, for the ads to be finished) with your phone. What if you reclaimed some white space in your life? What you may notice is that:

- You feel like you have more time
- You are more connected, present and mindful
- You are less distracted
- You feel less anxiety and stress
- You don't feel controlled by your phone.

It's a simple practice but allowing white space into your life can really help you feel much more present, connected with yourself and others and balanced. Resist the temptation to check your phone during those micro-gaps in your life spent waiting. Instead, look around and take in the moment.

Sleep

The purpose of sleep is to repair all our cells and rejuvenate our mind and body. Good quality sleep can boost your mood, balance your hormones and set you up in a healthy routine that will help combat illness and disease. Quite impressive, eh?

I've always found sleep a challenge. I'm a night owl and my anxiety can keep me up for hours each night, worrying about my to-do list. I am going to share the things I do that help me get enough sleep.

1. Wake up at the same time every day.

Even if you get to bed later, set your alarm to ring at the same time in the morning. You'll find you rise so much easier once your body clock is set.

2. Can't fall asleep? Try going to bed later.

This may sound counterproductive, but if you turn off the light too soon, you'll lie awake in bed for hours and feel increasingly frustrated. Go to bed later but still set your alarm for the same time each morning.

3. Struggle to wake up? Sleep with one of your blinds or curtains open or even slightly open.

The natural light will help you wake up more naturally.

4. Avoid drinking liquids for one to two hours before bed.

An interrupted night's sleep is often caused by a bathroom break. Drink liquids with dinner, but not too close to bed time. Many people recommend drinking chamomile tea (or similar) before bed to relax you; while this may help you fall asleep, waking up to go to the loo will disrupt your sleep.

5. Turn off the blue light from technology that can keep you alert and awake.

I'm guilty of streaming TV in bed before I sleep, but I find that reading a book before bed really helps my nervous system relax.

6. Charge your phone in another room.

Put your phone on charge from 8 pm onwards and then don't check it again. Not only does social media scrolling cause anxiety but the blue light from phones isn't helpful. Buy a separate alarm to wake you up.

7. Invest in a quality mattress.

You spend a third of your day in your bed, but I bet your car cost ten times the amount your mattress did. Invest in the best mattress you can afford.

8. Write down your worries.

Journalling or writing down your worries can help you stop replaying the same thoughts again and again. If I'm anxious, I'll do the reality checking exercise on page 123. If I have a mental to-do list, writing it down helps me forget about it until morning.

9. Check the temperature.
Make sure your room is well ventilated and there are extra blankets on hand in winter. Don't underestimate how important this is.

10. Practise meditation.
You don't need to become a yogi, but basic meditation exercises can help you reduce the chatter in your mind so you can fall asleep. I use mindful meditation apps. A simple body scan helps me a lot.

BODY SCAN EXERCISE

Lie on your back, arms by your side, and close your eyes. Make sure you're in a comfortable, relaxed position. Bring your attention to the limbs, one by one, working your way up your body. To start, become mindful of your toes and notice how they feel. Then bring your attention to your feet. Continue to work your way up your body, focusing on each body part until you reach the top of your head (if you're still awake by then!). This exercise should take about five to 10 minutes and will help bring you back into your body.

Alcohol
When you drink, your body prioritises processing of the alcohol over dipping into your fat stores for energy, so your metabolism slows. Plus, you lose self-control and your appetite increases with each tipple, so that a kebab (gyros), cheese platter or pizza slice seems more tempting. Furthermore, if you wake up the next day feeling a little weary, you're more likely to seek out comfort food to console you through your hangover.

Consistently drinking alcohol, especially when you're not in social situations, is often a form of numbing, a way of blocking out difficult emotions. Like food and exercise, developing a healthy relationship with alcohol is crucial. I drink alcohol, but I try to do so with balance; you can still have alcohol as part of a healthy diet, but less is best.

Reconsider your midweek drinking habits. I used to open a bottle of red wine during the week until I realised it was a habit. Now I generally don't drink alcohol during the week. That said, if I go out with friends midweek, I don't have a rule that says I can't have a glass of wine. I often volunteer to be the designated driver as this naturally curbs my drinking.

When you arrive at a party, ask for water first before having a glass of alcohol. Wait a while (say, 30 minutes) before having your first alcoholic drink. This doesn't sound like much, but this simple trick can help you drink less in this situation. In any case, you should drink plenty of water along with alcohol to help prevent dehydration.

Healthy glowing skin

Here's my simple guide for healthier skin.

Don't pick at your skin.
It's so tempting to pick at subtle imperfections on your skin but you always make them worse and it can lead to scarring. I learned this the hard way! Set a challenge not to pick your skin for a month and see how much better it looks.

Balance your hormones.
A lot of your skin health has to do with your hormones. Often, your hormones are out of your control—during puberty and menopause, for example—but avoiding low blood-sugar levels and hunger, reducing stress and getting enough sleep will help your hormones stabilise at other times.

Create consistency.
The more consistency you have, the more consistently healthy your skin will be. If you eat well for a few days, but binge on chocolate at the weekend, you might well get a breakout. But having a little chocolate each day is unlikely to make you break out.

Avoid getting ravenous or light-headed.
These are signs that your blood-sugar levels are low. The key to healthier skin is stable blood-sugar levels. Practise listening to your hunger and add satiating snacks if you're getting too hungry between meals.

Drink water.
Hydration is important for your skin health, among other things. Drink water and eat fresh fruit and vegetables. These also have the bonus of providing antioxidants that can help slow the ageing process, reduce inflammation and protect against breakouts.

Always wear sunscreen.
You can't undo skin damage. Whenever I exercise, no matter how early in the morning, I always put on sunscreen (and wear a hat). I use make-up with a sun protection factor (SPF) for an added barrier and keep sunscreen in my car.

Keep it real.
You can eat the most nutritious diet and your skin might still not reflect this. If your skin causes you trouble and you've tried strategies to improve it without success, don't blame yourself. There are so many environmental factors that are out of your control.

Speak to your doctor.
There's no need to struggle with acne, infections, psoriasis and eczema; these can all be treated.

feel amazing

Best foods for healthy skin

Try some of these delicious and nutritious foods to give your skin a great boost from the inside out.

Tomatoes – contain lycopene, which can protect your skin from sun damage. Chop tomatoes in a salad; add tomato paste to pasta, stews, soups and casseroles.

Dark chocolate – contains flavonoids, natural antioxidants that slow the signs of ageing. Add cacao to desserts or enjoy some dark chocolate with 70 per cent or higher cacao. Try the Chocolate chia pudding on page 149 for a chocolate hit.

Cauliflower – 100 g (3½ oz) of cauliflower will give you 77 per cent your recommended daily intake of vitamin C, which is an important antioxidant that can reduce inflammation and prevent pigmentation and discolouration. You also need vitamin C to produce collagen, for plumper skin.

Brazil nuts – packed with selenium, a nutrient powerhouse that helps maintain your skin's elastin, keeping your skin smooth and tight. Snack on a few brazil nuts or add them to grilled vegetables.

Plain Greek-style yoghurt – contains probiotics that will help fight inflammation related to acne, eczema and psoriasis. Enjoy yoghurt as a snack, add it to smoothies or serve with Lyndi's healthy home-made muesli on page 152.

Be realistic with your skin routine. Yeah, it's ideal to rinse your face, tone and moisturise twice a day, but if you can only manage to remove your make-up at night that's better than nothing. Done is better than perfect.

Salmon – heart-healthy omega–3 fats help combat inflammation, ideal if you suffer from skin problems such as acne, eczema or psoriasis. Try the Terrifically tasty teriyaki salmon on page 171.

Avocado – has plenty of 'healthy' fats. Adding this delicious ingredient to your meals will help balance your blood-sugar levels.

Oats – contain silica, which is great for firmer skin, thicker hair and stronger nails. Oats are low GI, which will also keep your blood-sugar levels more stable for better skin. Try the Get-up-and-go oats recipe on page 155.

Pepitas (pumpkin seeds) – contain zinc, which can help with wound healing and may help heal acne spots and marks. Add pepitas to your salads or muesli.

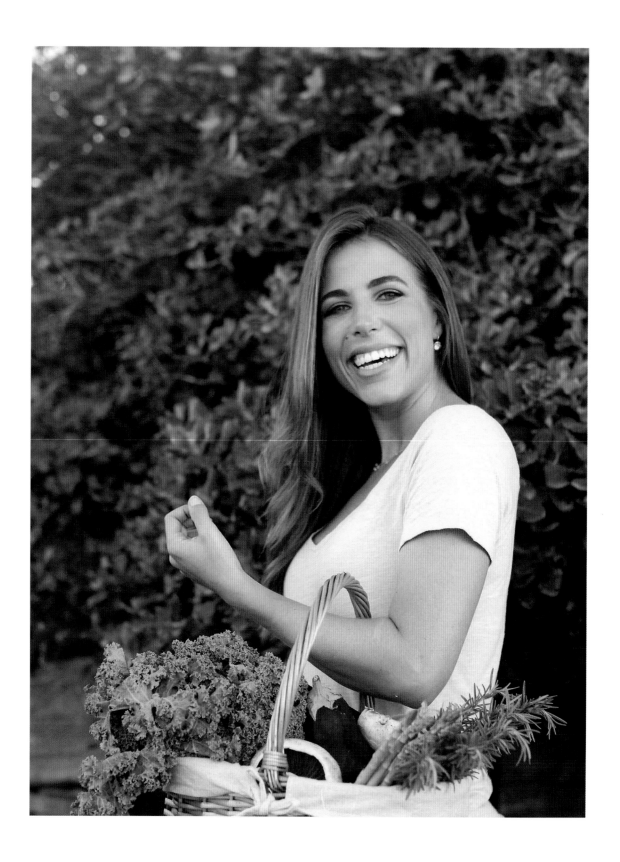

my recipes

The recipes in this book are designed to help you eat a more balanced diet that gives you energy. These are some of my favourite recipes, the foods I cook every day in my tiny kitchen, so I hope you enjoy them. My style of cooking is influenced by my culture, my community and my lack of a dishwasher: because no matter how good food tastes, who seriously wants to spend all day cooking and cleaning up? I don't. You'll find simple and easy-to-make recipes that you can prepare every day and still love. You don't need to spend a lot to make food taste great and fuel your body with all the wholesome stuff.
For more recipes and healthy inspiration, hop onto my website: lyndicohen.com/recipes.

Pantry essentials

These are the foods that are always stocked in my pantry that make it easy to make a healthy meal, even when there isn't any fresh food in the house. You'll also find many of these ingredients are used in the recipes in this book.

Grains and legumes

Chickpeas (garbanzo beans), tinned

Lentils or other beans of choice, tinned

Cannellini beans, tinned

Freekeh (found in the health-food aisle or wholegrains section)

Quinoa

Brown or black rice. I love the microwavable sachets for last minute meals

Self-raising flour, preferably wholemeal

Rolled (porridge) oats

Wholegrain bread. Sourdough is great, and the more seeds the better.

Plain (all-purpose) wholemeal flour

Pasta, wholemeal or legume

Dry ingredients

Seeds: pepitas (pumpkin seeds), sunflower seeds, linseeds (flaxseeds), sesame seeds, chia seeds

Nuts: cashews, almonds, peanuts, pistachios, walnuts, pecans, pine nuts

Dried coconut (flakes, desiccated, shredded)

Peanut butter or 100 per cent nut butter of choice

Cacao powder (not the same as cocoa powder)

Condiments

Extra virgin olive oil

Balsamic vinegar

Balsamic glaze

Tomato paste

Soy sauce or tamari (gluten-free soy sauce)

Fish sauce

Sesame oil (great for dressings and cooking)

Tahini

White wine vinegar

Sweet chilli sauce

Natural vanilla extract

Sweeteners

Maple syrup

Honey

Dates (dried and fresh Medjool)

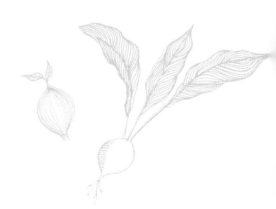

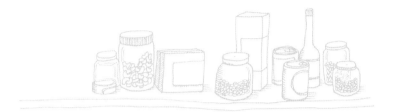

Herbs and spices

Turmeric

Paprika (sweet and smoked)

Cinnamon

Chilli flakes

Oregano

Cumin

Coriander (cilantro)

Sea salt

Garlic powder

Roasted vegetable seasoning

Za'atar (Middle Eastern herb and spice mix)

Other

Tins of tuna

Pickles. Great for snacking

Kalamata olives

Garlic

Vegetable stock

Onions, red and brown

Lemons and limes

Free-range eggs: boiled or scrambled eggs or
an omelette are fast and healthy meals that
will keep you feeling full.

Avocado

Tomatoes, tinned

Fridge favourites

ALL types of seasonal fruit

ALL types of seasonal vegetables

Full-fat Greek-style yoghurt

Milk of choice (I drink cow's milk, but drink
what makes you feel good)

Feta cheese. I like Danish.

Kimchi, kefir, kombucha and sauerkraut
(for gut health)

Fresh fish, chicken or lean red meat

A large jug of water

Hummus or dip. A dollop is great to add to
meals as a dressing. I make my own or buy
it ready made.

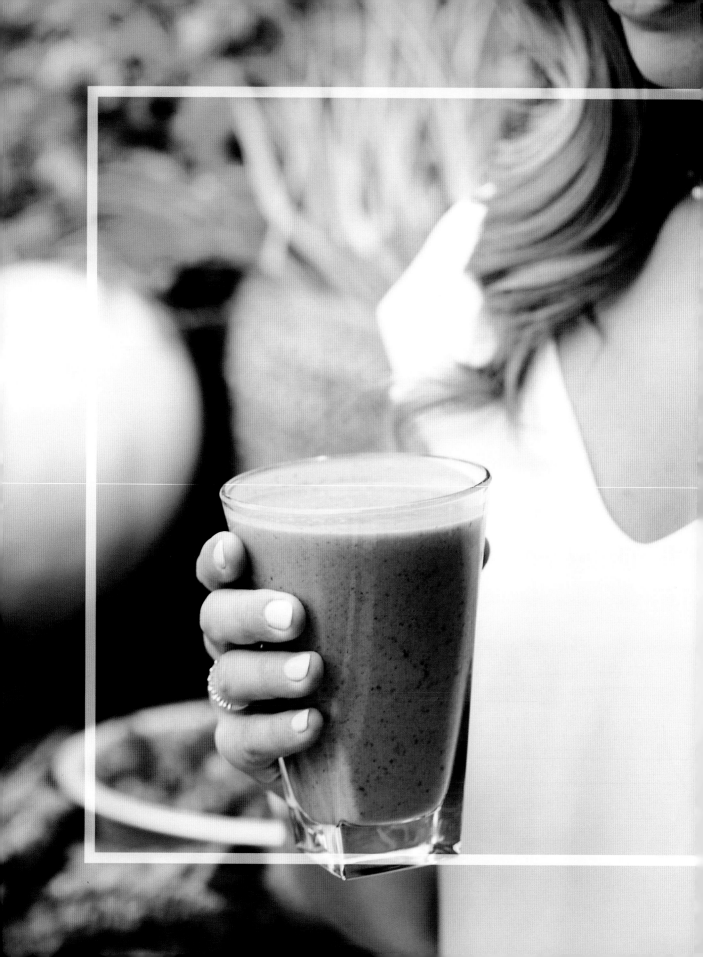

breakfast

There's not a lot of time in the morning to whip up a gourmet breakfast, so this is quite simply an everyday option, filled with superfoods, that will take just five minutes to prepare. It's a perfect balance of slow-burning carbs, lean protein and 'healthy' fats, plus you'll fuel up with all the goodness of two serves of vegetables before you've even started your day!

Big breakfast bowl

PREP TIME: 3 MINUTES

COOKING TIME: 2 MINUTES

SERVES 1

1 teaspoon extra virgin olive oil

2 free-range eggs

1 piece of grainy bread, toasted

½ cup (75 g) cherry tomatoes, chopped (or 1 large tomato, chopped)

1 handful of spinach leaves

¼ avocado

1 tablespoon pepitas (pumpkin seeds) or sunflower seeds

1 teaspoon balsamic glaze (see tip)

Preheat a frying pan to medium–high heat and add the olive oil. Whisk the eggs in bowl, add to the pan with a pinch of salt and stir until scrambled.

Arrange the eggs with the remaining ingredients in a bowl and drizzle with the balsamic glaze to serve.

Tips

- *If you have other vegetables in the fridge—such as mushrooms, asparagus, baked vegies or even cucumber—use them up and get creative. Once you get into a habit of eating vegies for breakfast, and you realise how good it makes you feel, it soon feels normal to eat a salad to start the day.*
- *Balsamic glaze is made from balsamic vinegar, sweetened and cooked until it's reduced to a thick syrup. If you can't find it in the supermarket, make your own or just use balsamic vinegar and a little honey instead.*
- *Use gluten-free bread if you want to make this gluten free. Swap the eggs for tofu to make it vegan.*

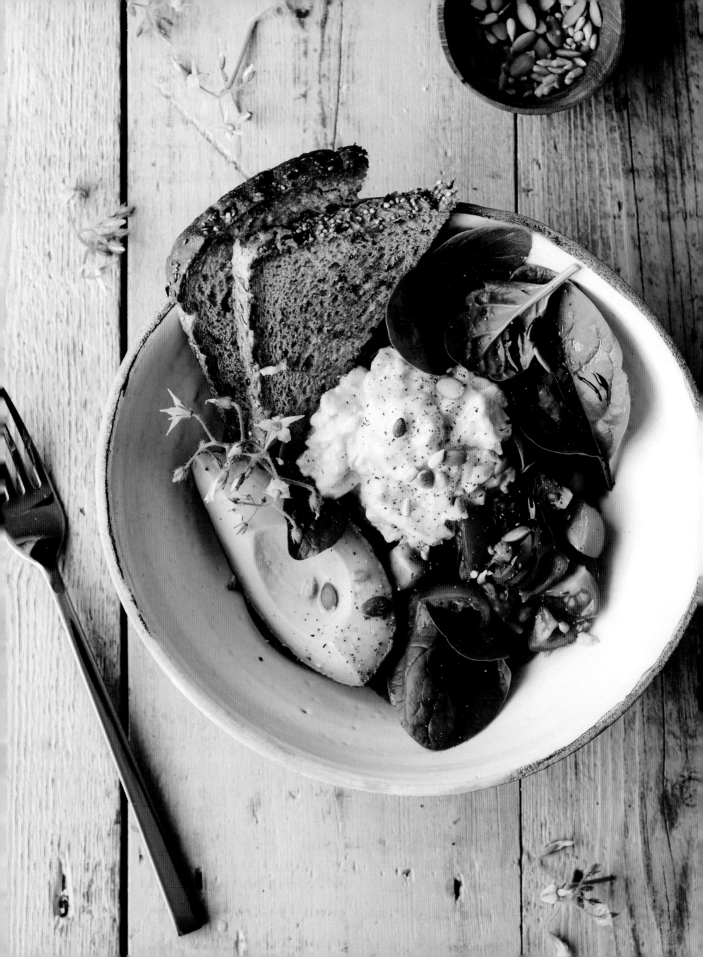

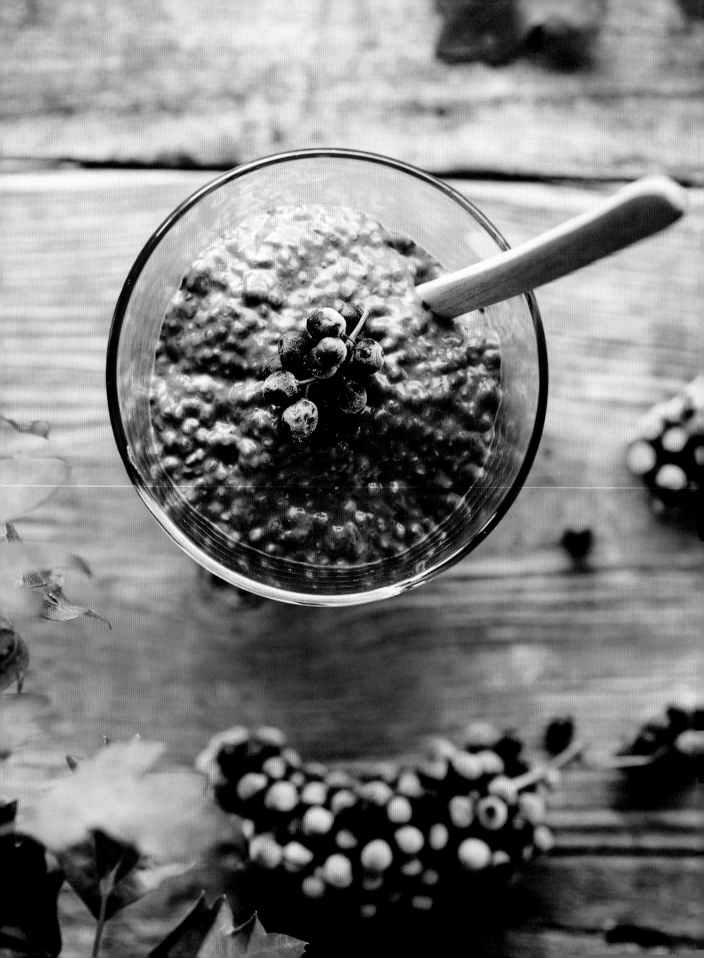

I won't lie to you: chocolate is my favourite food so chocolate for breakfast is my idea of fun. Luckily, this is a seriously good-for-you breakfast or snack. It's delicious and loaded with fibre.

Chocolate chia pudding

Put all of the ingredients in a jar or container with a lid and shake to combine.

Refrigerate until set, ideally overnight.

PREP TIME: 5 MINS
SETTING TIME: 2+ HOURS

SERVES 1

3½ tablespoons chia seeds
1 cup (250 ml) milk
2 tablespoons cacao powder
1½ tablespoons maple syrup
1 teaspoon vanilla essence
⅛ teaspoon salt

Tips

- *You can prepare this chocolate chia pudding ahead of time, keep it in the fridge and take it to work easily.*
- *Play around by adding other flavours you love, such as peanut butter, mashed banana or cinnamon. I love dairy but use a nut milk to make it dairy free or vegan if that feels good!*
- *Maple syrup is a natural sugar source, but let's be real: it's still sugar. That doesn't mean it's 'bad' for you or should be banned from your diet (you really can eat everything in moderation, pinky promise) but this recipe isn't 'sugar-free' as some people might claim. #keepitreal Either way, enjoy it wholeheartedly.*

everyday option • gluten free • low gi • high fibre • heart healthy • healthy ageing • diabetes friendly

A delicious snack or light breakfast, this power smoothie is beautifully balanced and filling. I'm kind of obsessed, in a healthy way.

Energy-boosting green smoothie

PREP TIME: 5 MINUTES

SERVES 1

1 cup (45 g) baby spinach leaves
1 cup (250 ml) milk
1 tablespoon 100% nut butter
1 frozen banana
1 fresh medjool date, pitted
½ cup ice cubes

Combine all of the ingredients in a blender and blitz for 30 seconds or until it has a creamy texture.

Tips

- Use the milk that makes you feel good, whether that's full-fat or low-fat dairy or nut milks to make it dairy free or vegan.
- Be sure to peel and slice your banana before freezing so you don't break your blender.
- If your machine can't chop ice, simply add a few cubes before you drink it.

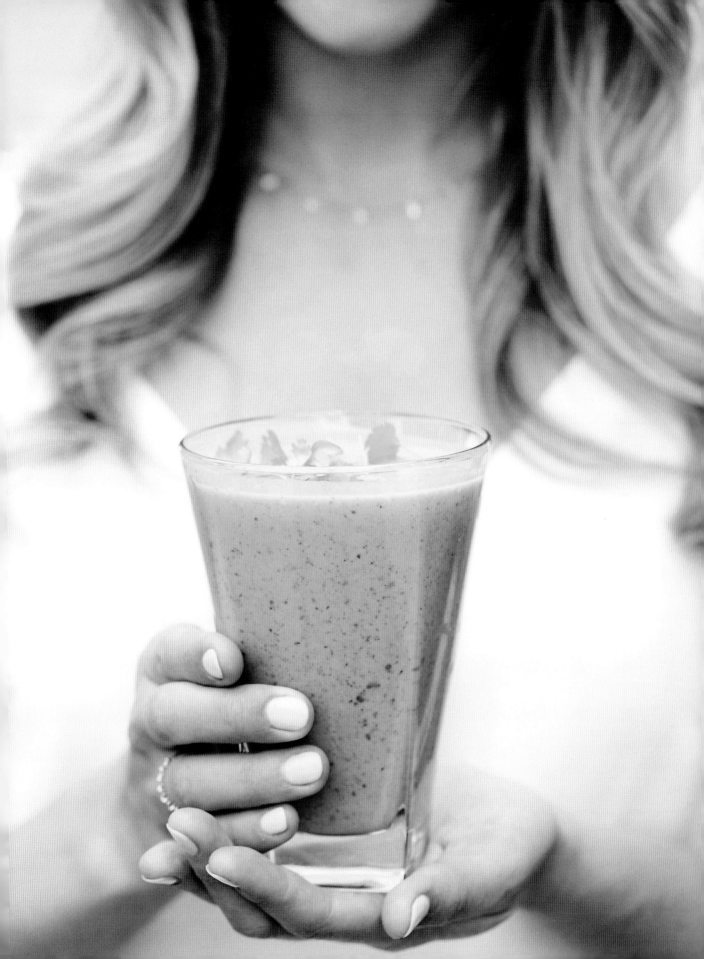

You'll be surprised how quick and easy it is to make your own breakfast cereal (and how good it will make your house smell). This muesli will keep in the fridge for up to a month. Freeze some if you have extra. Serve with Greek-style yoghurt and fresh fruit. Play around with the flavours. You can add coconut flakes, chia seeds or cinnamon and use apricots or raisins instead of dates.

Lyndi's healthy home-made muesli

PREP TIME: 5 MINUTES
COOKING TIME: 35 MINUTES

**MAKES 1.5 KG (3 LB 5 OZ);
SERVES 30 (ABOUT ⅓ CUP)**

1½ cups (750 g) rolled (porridge)
   oats
2 cups chopped nuts (such as
   1 cup almonds, ½ cup crushed
   peanuts and ½ cup cashews)
2 cups mixed seeds (such as
   1 cup sunflower seeds +
   1 cup pepitas)
3 tablespoons maple syrup
3 tablespoons extra virgin olive oil
1 cup (160 g) chopped pitted dates

Preheat the oven to 180°C (350°F). Line two or three large baking trays with baking paper.

Mix together the oats, nuts and seeds in a large bowl. Slowly drizzle some of the maple syrup and olive oil into the mix and stir. Season with a pinch of salt. Repeat this process until the mixture is evenly (and lightly) coated.

Spread the mixture on lined baking trays and bake for 30–35 minutes until golden brown and toasted. You may want to stir the muesli halfway through the cooking time to ensure even toasting.

Remove from the oven and allow the muesli to cool on the trays. Add the dates and store in an airtight container.

Tips

- *This muesli won't taste sweet or hold together in clusters like store-bought varieties.*
- *I buy a packet of mixed seeds and nuts.*
- *If you're gluten intolerant, buy certified gluten-free oats. Not all oats are gluten free.*
- *When grocery shopping, check the three Cs: if a breakfast cereal says 'crispy', 'crunchy' or 'clusters', it's a dead giveaway that the cereal has quite a bit of sugar and fat added to give it the crunchy texture. Solution? Check the ingredients list or make your own.*

Who really has loads of time in the morning? Toast is perfectly nutritious, especially with some satiating toppings. Of all breads, I love wholegrain and brown the most, particularly if it's sourdough. The darker the colour and the grainier the texture, the better.

Tight-on-time toast, four ways

Toast the bread in your toaster or under the grill (broiler) in the oven. Pile on the toppings of your choice and serve.

PREP TIME: 5 MINUTES
COOKING TIME: 5 MINUTES

SERVES 1

1 slice wholegrain sourdough
   bread

AVO CUDDLE TO FEEL FETA
¼ avocado
1 tablespoon crumbled feta cheese
1 pinch of dried chilli flakes

RICOTTA HONEY
¼ cup (60 g) fresh ricotta cheese
1 teaspoon honey, or balsamic
   glaze
2–3 strawberries, sliced (optional)

**GO BANANAS, GO NUTS,
   GO CRAZY!**
1 tablespoon nut butter
½ banana, sliced
½ teaspoon ground cinnamon

HUMMUS FETA
2 tablespoons hummus
1 tablespoon crumbled feta cheese
1 pinch of dried chilli flakes

Tips

- *Serve your toast with vegies, such as a punnet of cherry tomatoes, a handful of baby spinach or some sautéed mushrooms.*
- *Adding fresh fruit is lovely. Add sliced strawberries in early summer or slices of persimmon in autumn.*
- *Sourdough is the least processed type of bread, containing few ingredients and lots of fibre.*
- *If you're using a packaged bread, check the ingredients list to be sure there isn't added sugar. Many breads have added sugar, which is confusing and unnecessary.*
- *Use gluten-free toast if you want to make it gluten free. Some of the options are also nut free and dairy free.*

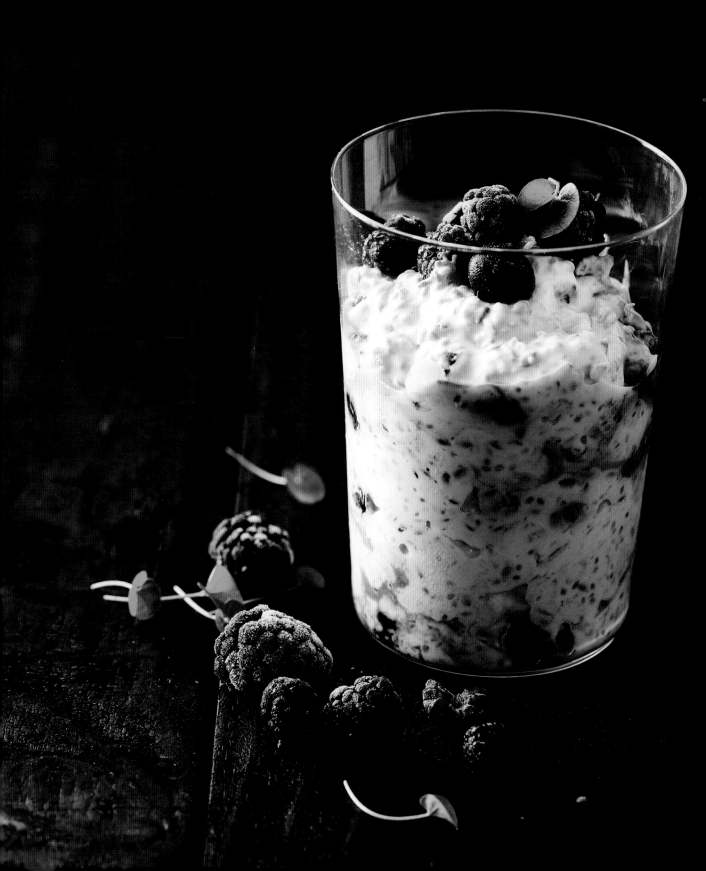

This is a great basic recipe because it's so simple: it means you can truly listen to your hunger, as this pot of goodness can be taken with you to be eaten when your hunger grows. Make a whole batch of these oat pots so you've got some delicious healthy meals ready ahead of a busy week.

Get-up-and-go overnight oats

Stir together the milk, yoghurt, oats, honey, vanilla and mixed seeds in a jar. Top with the frozen berries (if using) and let it soak in the fridge for at least 3 hours or preferably overnight.

PREP TIME: 5 MINUTES (PLUS OVERNIGHT SOAKING)

SERVES 1

⅓ cup (80 ml) milk
⅓ cup (95 g) Greek-style yoghurt
⅓ cup (35 g) rolled (porridge) oats
2 teaspoons honey
1 teaspoon natural vanilla extract
2 tablespoons mixed seeds,
    such as linseeds (flaxseeds),
    sunflower seeds, pepitas
    (pumpkin seeds) and chia seeds
⅓ cup (45 g) frozen berries
    (optional)

Tips

- *You can experiment and swap the honey for half a shredded apple or 1 tablespoon of raisins or currants, add a handful of chopped nuts or play around and add different seasonal fruit. If you don't have frozen fruit, fresh chopped or a bit of dried fruit is great.*
- *Look for a Greek-style yoghurt with probiotics.*
- *Use certified gluten-free oats if you need to make it gluten free and nut milk or coconut yoghurt to make it dairy free and vegan.*

Oats, berries and Greek-style yoghurt are three everyday superfoods. Combined with the longlasting energy from banana and the calcium and protein from the milk, this is one super healthy way to start your day. Don't have much time in the morning? Serve this as a smoothie instead. Kids will think it's a strawberry thickshake!

Berry good breakfast bowl

PREP TIME: 5 MINUTES

SERVES 1

¼ cup (25 g) rolled (porridge) oats

½ cup (125 ml) milk

1 frozen banana

½ cup (70 g) frozen berries

⅓ cup (95 g) Greek-style yoghurt

1 medjool date, pitted

Combine all of the ingredients in a blender and blitz for 1 minute or until the texture is creamy. Pour into a bowl to serve.

Tips

- Top with a handful of frozen berries and Lyndi's healthy home-made muesli (see page 152).
- Use certified gluten-free oats if you need to make it gluten free and nut milk or coconut yoghurt to make it dairy free and vegan.

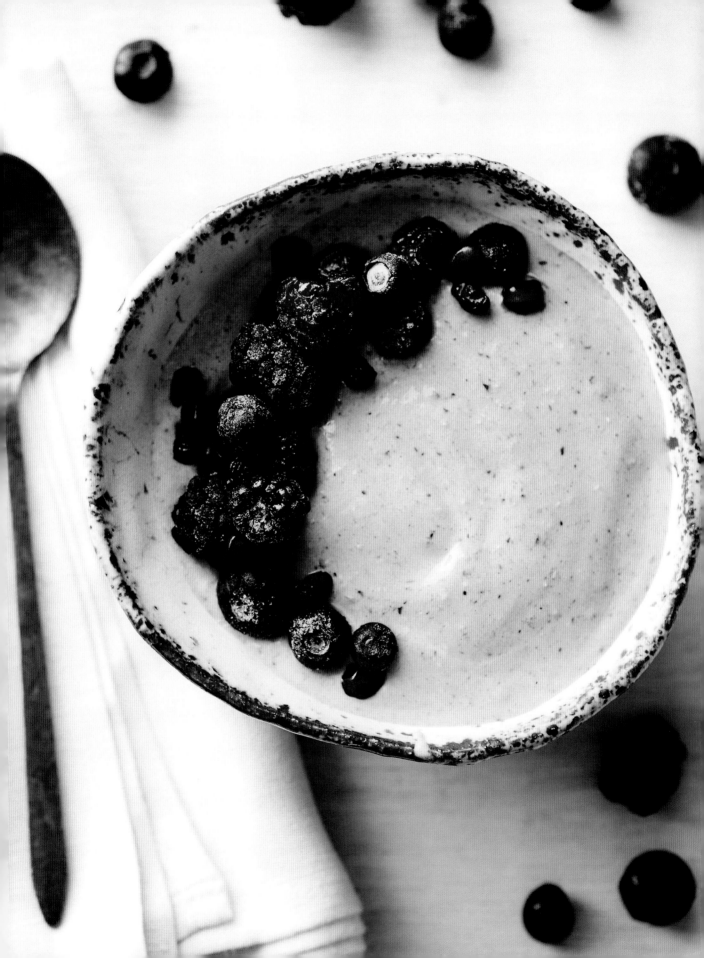

Warm, comforting and oh so good for you, this nourishing porridge is Goldilocks approved because it's beautifully balanced and tastes just right. It's fibre-rich and protein-packed to keep you satisfied for longer, your gut healthy and your cravings at bay. You can't help but feel good when you start your day with this recipe.

Goldilocks's favourite power porridge

PREP TIME: 2 MINUTES

COOKING TIME: 5 MINUTES

SERVES 1

⅓ cup (35 g) rolled (porridge) oats

½ cup (125 ml) milk

1 tablespoon chia seeds

1 tablespoon of pepitas (pumpkin seeds), sunflower seeds or linseeds (flaxseeds)

½ teaspoon vanilla extract

¼ teaspoon ground cinnamon

Put all of the ingredients in a small saucepan with ⅓ cup (80 ml) of water and bring it to the boil. Stir over medium heat for 5 minutes, until the oats are creamy.

Transfer to a small bowl to serve.

Tips

- Serve with 1 teaspoon of nut butter, diced dates or ½ a banana and some seeds.
- Use certified gluten-free oats if you need to make it gluten free and milk alternative or coconut yoghurt to make it dairy free and vegan.

This is my go-to juice that I have pretty much every morning after I exercise, but it's also perfect the day after (or before) drinking alcohol, to boost your nutrient levels and balance out the bender.

Post-bender booster green juice

Put all of the ingredients into a juicer or blender and process for 1 minute or until combined. If using a blender, strain into a glass to serve.

PREP TIME: 10 MINUTES

SERVES: 1

1 cucumber
½ lemon, peeled
1 cup (45 g) baby spinach leaves
1 cup water
1 teaspoon honey or maple syrup
1 cm (⅜ inch) piece of ginger, peeled
¼ cup (5 g) fresh mint leaves
1 green apple

Tips

- *Got coconut water? Swap the water and honey for one cup of coconut water.*
- *I don't own a juicer, so I blend the ingredients and strain through a coffee plunger, a sieve or muslin (cheesecloth). It works a treat!*
- *If you love the pulp, there is no need to strain this.*
- *Use maple syrup instead of honey to make a vegan option.*

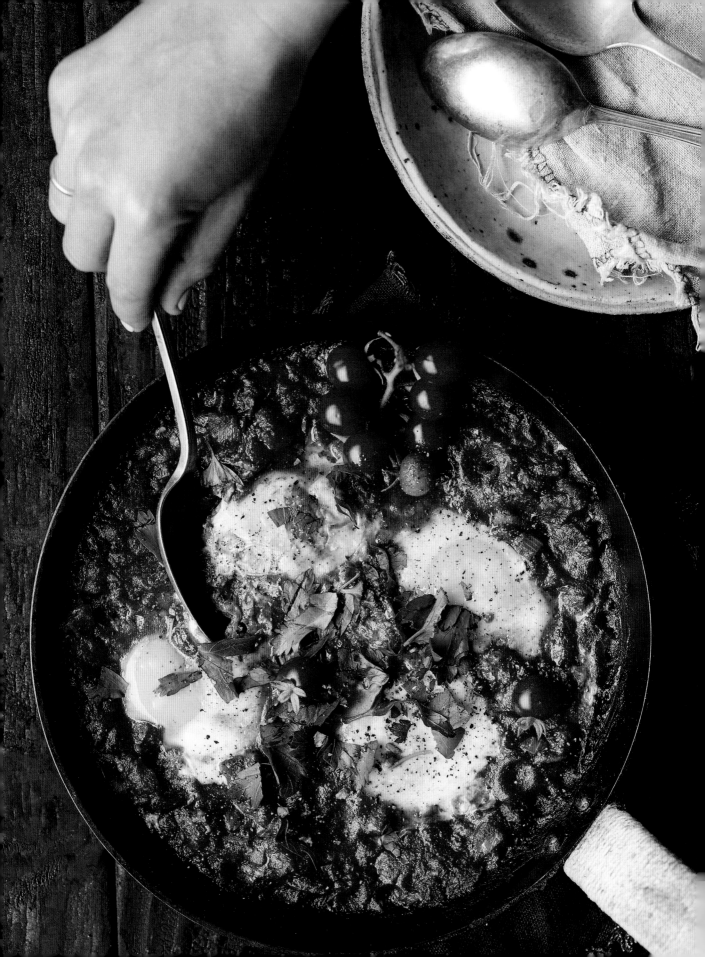

These delicious baked eggs (based on the traditional shakshuka) are a family favourite, and a fantastic way to get another serve of vegies into your day. You don't have to leave this dish for breakfasts only: I love it at dinner time too. Serve it straight from the skillet or frying pan for that extra 'wow' factor.

Easy like a Sunday morning eggs

Heat the olive oil in a large frying pan over medium heat. Add the onion and cook for 5 minutes or until soft.

Add the tomatoes, tomato paste, garlic, cumin, chilli flakes and salt. Add a little water if it becomes too thick. Cook for 10 minutes.

Make little wells in the tomato mixture and break the eggs into the wells. Cover the pan with a lid and simmer for 5 minutes until the egg whites are cooked but the yolks are still soft.

Meanwhile, toast the bread.

To serve, scatter the parsley over the top and scoop the eggs and tomato mixture out of the pan onto the toast.

PREP TIME: 5 MINUTES
COOKING TIME: 20 MINUTES

SERVES 4

1 tablespoon extra virgin olive oil
1 small brown onion, finely
    chopped
two 400 g (14 oz) tins chopped
    tomatoes
1 tablespoon tomato paste
3 garlic cloves, crushed
2 teaspoons ground cumin
½ teaspoon dried chilli flakes
½ teaspoon salt
4 free-range eggs
4 slices grainy sourdough bread
2 tablespoons chopped parsley,
    to serve

Tips

• *If you love this recipe but don't have time on weekdays, you can make lots of the tomato sauce (up to the second step) and store the mixture in the fridge or freezer. Then simply heat it in the frying pan in the morning and add the eggs. This is a great breakfast if you like to go camping.*
• *If you love mushrooms, add a cup of chopped mushrooms with the tomatoes. Like it hot? Add an extra ½ teaspoon of chilli flakes for a delicious warm heat.*
• *Use gluten-free toast if you want to make it gluten free.*

I wouldn't recommend this for breakfast; it's more of a mid-morning snack. I'm not a fan of protein powders, as they are often so processed they no longer resemble the food they are made from. If you're like me and want a 'real food' option for a protein bar, these are great. Pack a bar in your lunchbox for a high-protein boost.

Natural chocolate protein bar

PREP TIME: 5 MINUTES

SERVES 5

½ cup (50 g) rolled (porridge) oats
½ cup (80 g) almonds, skin on
2 tablespoons cacao powder
¼ cup (40 g) chia seeds
¼ teaspoon salt
6 fresh dates, pitted
2 tablespoons water

Line an 11 x 21 cm (4¼ x 8¼ inch) loaf tin with baking paper and set aside.

Put all of the ingredients in a food processor. Blitz until roughly chopped, then spread the mixture in the prepared tin. Press down firmly on the mixture and refrigerate for 20 minutes.

Slice crossways into 4 cm (1½ inch) wide bars.

Tips

- *With more than 6 g (¼ oz) of natural plant-based protein per serve, plus a whopping amount of gut-friendly fibre, these bars are a fantastic option for a healthy snack after exercise, when you get hungry in the afternoon or for kids as a nutritious after-school snack.*
- *Use gluten-free oats if you're allergic or intolerant.*
- *Add a drizzle of maple syrup if you want it a little sweeter.*

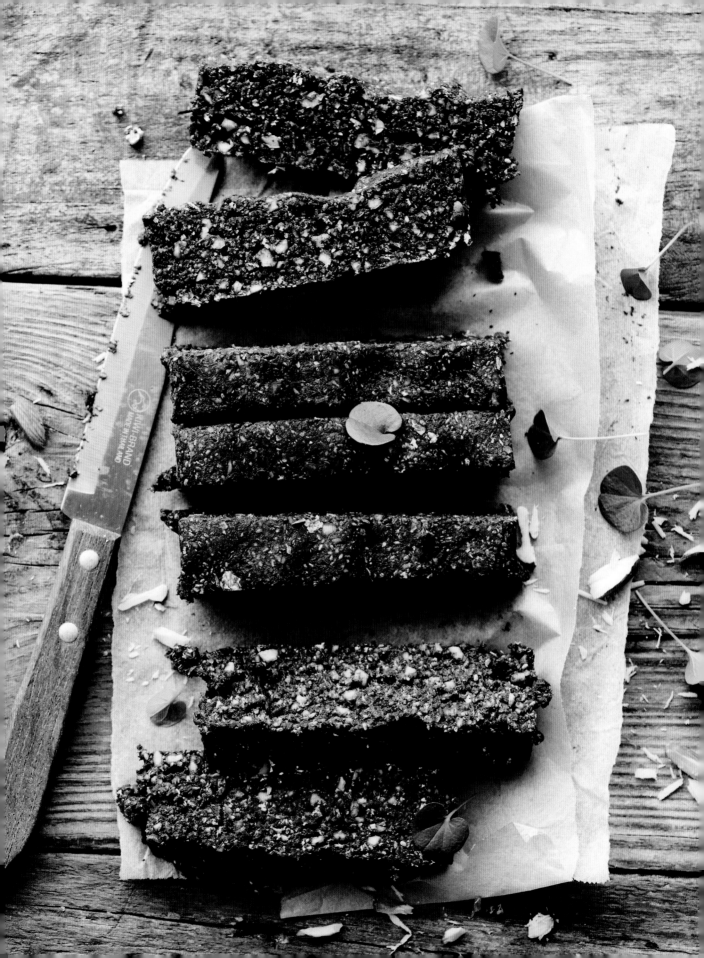

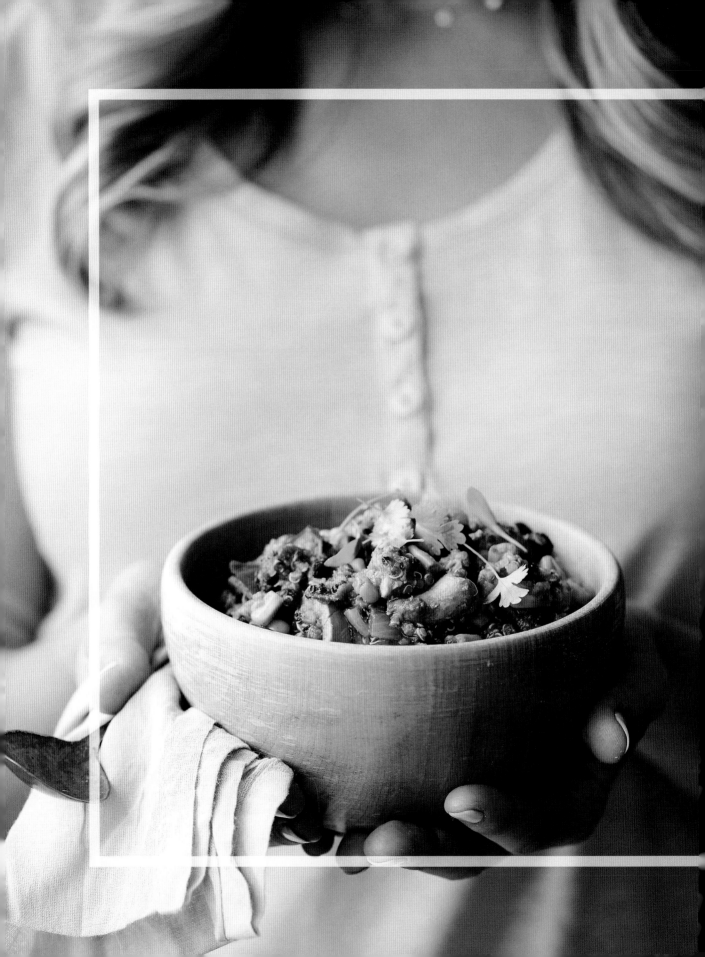

main meals

I would never, ever give up pasta forever, so why not make it fit into my healthy, balanced life? I sneak vegies into my sauce and love to serve my vegie-full bolognese with salad and pasta. If you want more vegies, dish up half the bowl with pasta and the other side with whatever vegies are around: spiralised carrots or zucchini (courgettes), shredded lettuce leaves, steamed vegies.

Vegie-full beef bolognese with real spaghetti

PREP TIME: 2 MINUTES
COOKING TIME: 25 MINUTES

SERVES 4–6

1 brown onion, coarsely chopped

1 carrot, coarsely chopped

250 g (9 oz) button mushrooms

2 tablespoons extra virgin olive oil

2 tablespoons tomato paste
   (tomato concentrate)

2 garlic cloves

1/2 teaspoon salt

400 g (14 oz) minced beef

two 400 g (14 oz) tins of chopped
   tomatoes

2 tablespoons balsamic vinegar

500 g (1 lb 2 oz) wholemeal
   spaghetti (gluten-free
   if desired)

handful of basil leaves, to serve

Put the onion, carrot and mushrooms in a food processor and blitz until finely chopped. Alternatively, finely chop all the vegetables.

Heat a large saucepan over medium-high heat and add the olive oil. When the oil is hot, add the chopped vegies and cook for 5 minutes, stirring, until caramelised.

Add the tomato paste, garlic and salt, stir well, and cook for a further 3 minutes.

Add the beef, breaking up lumps, and stir it through the vegetables. Cook for 5 minutes.

Add the tomatoes and balsamic vinegar and cook for a further 10 minutes.

Meanwhile, cook the spaghetti according to the packet directions. Divide the spaghetti between plates and top with the sauce. Serve with fresh basil.

Tips

- If you have fussy eaters, blitz the vegies a little finer so they are more hidden.
- This bolognese is ideal for easy meal prep, so whip up a whole batch (or two or three!) ahead of a busy week. Freeze the extras.
- The longer you cook bolognese, the tastier it becomes; if you have time, simmer it for an hour in total (check regularly and add a little water if necessary to ensure it doesn't burn).

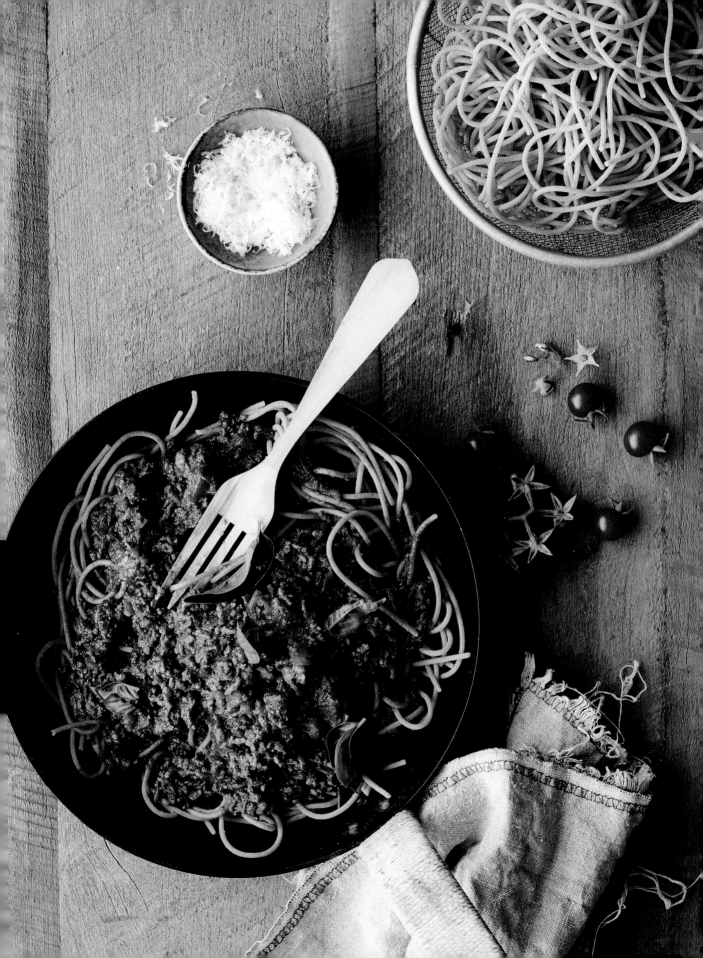

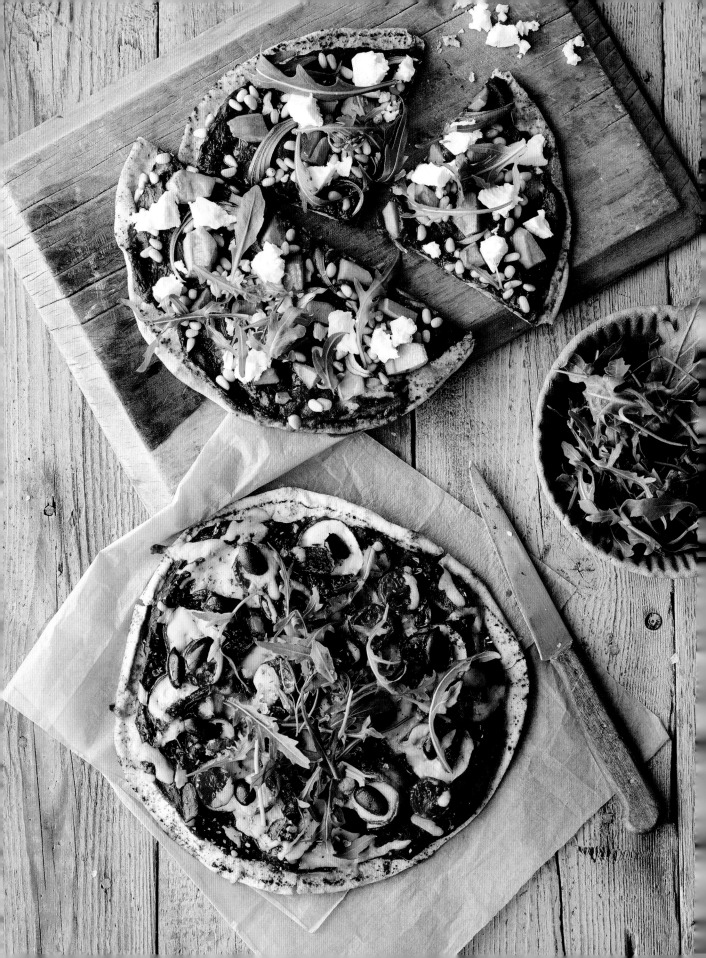

Who wants to live without pizza? Flatbread makes the perfect, crispy base for fresh pizza when you don't have a professional pizza oven.

Family favourite flatbread pizzas

Preheat the oven to 180°C (350°F).

Mix the tomato paste with the oregano and garlic. Spread the tomato paste evenly on one side of each flatbread round.

Add your preferred toppings. Bake for 10 minutes until golden brown. Add the feta cheese, if using, and serve with the rocket leaves scattered over the top or on the side as a salad.

PREP TIME: 10 MINUTES
COOKING TIME: 10 MINUTES

SERVES 4

500 g (1 lb 2 oz) jar of tomato
    paste (tomato concentrate)
1½ tablespoons dried oregano
2 garlic cloves, finely chopped
4–6 wholemeal flatbread rounds
rocket (arugula) leaves, to serve

VEGIE-LOVERS TOPPING
1 zucchini (courgette), sliced
¼ cup (40 g) sun-dried tomatoes
¼ cup (40 g) kalamata olives,
    pitted and halved
½ cup (75 g) cherry tomatoes,
    halved
2 button mushrooms, sliced
2 cups (250 g) shredded
    mozzarella cheese

SWEET PUMPKIN TOPPING
¼ cup chopped pumpkin (squash)
¼ red onion, sliced
2 tablespoons pine nuts
⅓ cup (50 g) crumbled feta cheese
    (add after cooking)

Tips

- *If you've got fussy eaters in your family, this recipe is great because everyone can make their own pizza. Serve the toppings buffet-style and challenge the family to make their own combinations.*
- *Opt for a gluten-free flatbread base if you're intolerant or allergic.*
- *Can't have too much lactose? Parmesan has a much lower lactose content than other cheeses. Parmesan is also a lot stronger in flavour so you need less for a cheesy hit.*
- *Swap the pine nuts for pepitas (pumpkin seeds) if you prefer them.*

Talk about comfort food. Meatballs have it all, especially when you sneak in more vegies. If you have fussy eaters, blend the vegetables up thoroughly or leave the parsley and use as a garnish instead.

Mumma's meatballs

PREP TIME: 5 MINUTES
COOKING TIME: 10 MINUTES

SERVES 6 (MAKES 24 MEATBALLS)

200 g (7 oz) button mushrooms

1 onion

2 garlic cloves

2 teaspoons smoked paprika

1 cup loosely packed (20 g) parsley
   leaves

1 zucchini (courgette)

2 teaspoons ground cumin

1–2 chillies

1 teaspoon salt

500 g (1 lb 2 oz) minced lamb
   or beef

½ cup (30 g) fresh breadcrumbs

½ cup (45 g) grated or shaved
   parmesan cheese

1 egg

1 tablespoon of extra virgin olive
   oil

1–2 tablespoons pine nuts
   (optional)

Put the mushrooms, onion, garlic, paprika, parsley, zucchini, cumin, chillies and salt into food processor and blitz to a coarse texture. Transfer to a medium bowl. Add the minced meat, breadcrumbs, parmesan and egg and use your hands to mix the ingredients well, then form into golf ball–size balls.

Heat the olive oil in a large frying pan over medium–high heat. Fry the meatballs for 8–10 minutes, turning regularly to brown on all sides. Add the pine nuts to the pan in the last two minutes of cooking, if using.

Serve meatballs with Cheeky tzatziki (see page 210), wholemeal pita bread and Quinoa pomegranate tabouleh (see page 192).

Tips

- You can make your own breadcrumbs by blitzing up your favourite day-old bread in a food processor; if using ready-made dry breadcrumbs, use half the quantity.
- You can also add herbs like coriander (cilantro) or mint.
- Use gluten-free breadcrumbs or quinoa flakes if you're allergic or intolerant.
- Prefer to bake these? Preheat the oven to 200°C (400°F). Set the balls on a baking tray lined with baking paper and cook for 25 minutes. Turn the oven to grill (broil) for the final 2 minutes.

This teriyaki salmon recipe makes me happy. It's damn delicious, but don't take my word for it. Serve it with wholegrains such as quinoa or brown rice and loads of vegies for a beautifully balanced meal that the whole clan will love.

Terrifically tasty teriyaki salmon

Combine the soy sauce, maple syrup, olive and sesame oils, ginger and garlic in a shallow bowl. Add the salmon fillets and marinate for at least 5 minutes (the longer the better).

Heat a frying pan over medium-high heat. Place the salmon in the pan with 2 tablespoons of marinade. Cook on one side for 3 minutes then turn over. Add the rest of the marinade, cover with a lid and cook for a further 3 minutes. Swirl the pan to make sure sauce isn't burning.

Top with sesame seeds (if using), to serve.

PREP TIME: 5 MINUTES
COOKING TIME: 6 MINUTES

SERVES 2

3 tablespoons soy sauce
3 tablespoons maple syrup
2 tablespoons extra virgin olive oil
1 teaspoon sesame oil
1 teaspoon freshly grated ginger
1–2 garlic cloves, crushed
2 salmon fillets, 125 g (4½ oz) each
1 teaspoon sesame seeds (optional), to serve

Tips

- You can also make an entire meal using this marinade. Simply double the marinade recipe and lay the salmon fillets, along with vegetables such as broccoli, capsicum, carrot and snow peas, on a baking tray lined with baking paper. Bake for 15–20 minutes at 200°C (400°F). You'll have dinner ready in a jiffy... and only one tray to clean up. Get the full recipe at lyndicohen.com/recipes
- Use tamari (gluten-free soy sauce) instead of soy sauce if you're sensitive to gluten.
- This marinade is also great with chicken (thighs work best). Either grill in a frying pan or bake in the oven until cooked.

Boy oh boy, I love this recipe. To be honest, this isn't authentic pad Thai, but it's seriously good so I'm hoping you won't mind too much. I've swapped rice noodles for zucchini (courgette) noodles, not because noodles are unhealthy (they aren't!), but it's a brilliant way to get more veg into your day. #crowding

Zucchini noodle pad Thai

PREP TIME: 15 MINUTES
COOKING TIME: 15 MINUTES

SERVES 4

¼ cup (35 g) peanuts, chopped
1 tablespoon extra virgin olive oil
400 g (14 oz) chicken stir-fry strips
1–2 red chillies, chopped
3 spring onions (scallions), chopped
1 handful coriander (cilantro),
    leaves picked and stems chopped
250 g (9 oz) mushrooms, chopped
2 eggs, whisked
5 zucchini (courgettes), spiralised
    or shaved into ribbons

PAD THAI SAUCE
2 tablespoons soy sauce or tamari
    (gluten-free soy sauce)
2 tablespoons sweet chilli sauce
2 tablespoons peanut butter
1 tablespoon honey
2–3 garlic cloves
¼ cup (60 ml) water

Combine all of the ingredients for the sauce in a small bowl, mix well and set aside.

Heat a frying pan over high heat. Toast the peanuts for 2–3 minutes. Remove from the pan and set aside.

Heat the olive oil in the pan, add the chicken and cook for 3 minutes. Add the chilli, spring onion and chopped coriander stems and stir-fry for 2 minutes.

Add the mushrooms and stir-fry for a further 2 minutes. Add the egg and stir-fry for 2 minutes more. Add the zucchini and cook for a further 2 minutes. Add the sauce and cook for 2 minutes more.

Divide between bowls or plates and scatter with the coriander leaves and toasted peanuts.

Tips

- *You'll need a spiraliser for this recipe, which you can buy from most homewares shops.*
- *If you love a mild to medium heat, use two chillies with the seeds. Otherwise stick to one and remove the seeds for an even milder flavour. You can always add dried chilli flakes later if you want more heat.*
- *This sauce is great for other stir-fries too.*
- *Toasted and crushed walnuts (or other nuts) work equally as well as peanuts.*
- *You can add colour with carrot noodles (add them before the eggs to ensure they are thoroughly cooked).*

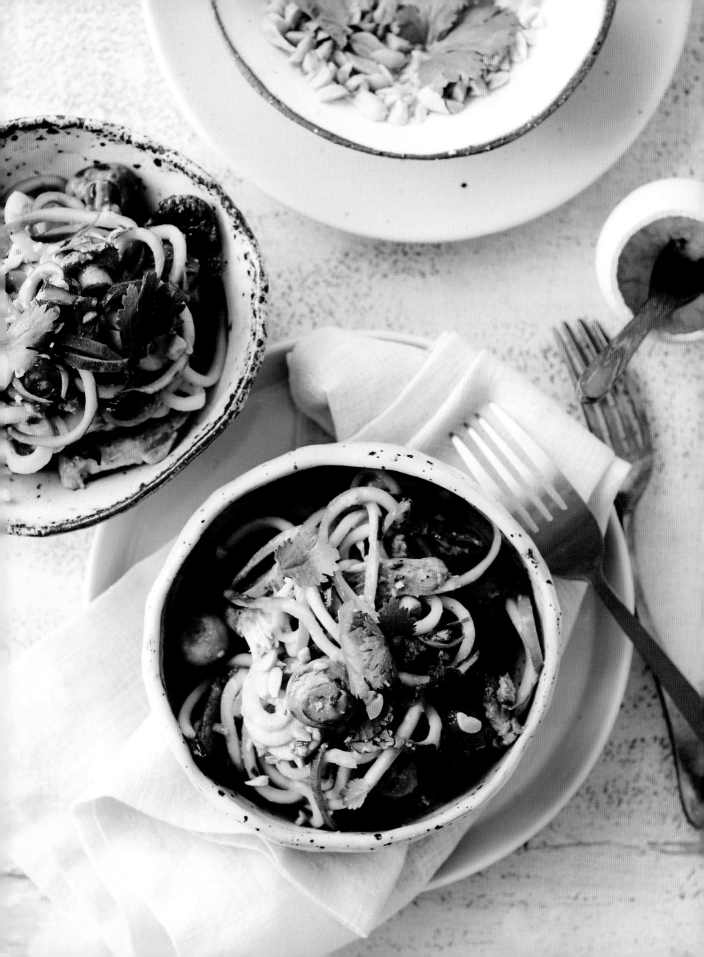

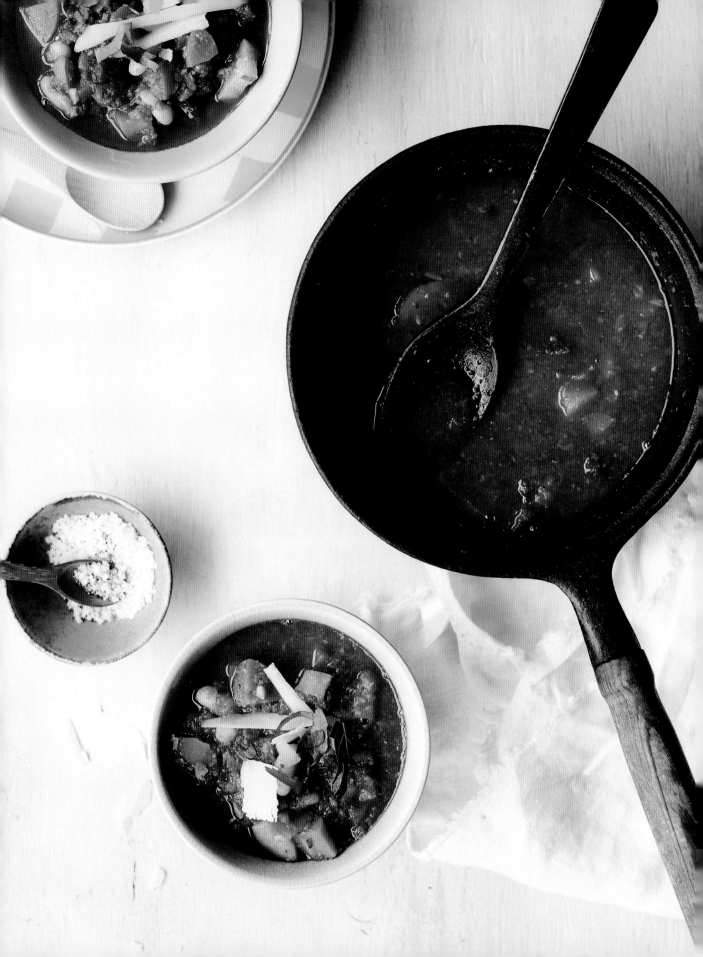

everyday option • gluten free • vegetarian • low gi • high fibre
heart healthy • healthy ageing • diabetes friendly • nut free

Minestrone is known as peasant food but this humble soup has endured through the centuries and remains one of the most nutritious meals there is.

Nonna's minestrone

Blitz the onion, 2 carrots, 2 zucchini, the celery and parsley in a food processor until finely chopped.

Heat the olive oil in a large saucepan or stockpot over high heat. Add the chopped vegetables and sauté for 10 minutes or until golden.

Add the tomato, tomato paste, garlic and cumin and simmer for 5 minutes.

Coarsely chop the remaining zucchini and carrot and add to the pan with the stock. Boil, then simmer, covered, for at least 20 minutes and up to 3 hours.

Add the cannellini beans and pepper in the last 10 minutes of cooking.

Ladle into bowls and serve topped with shaved parmesan and chopped parsley leaves.

PREP TIME: 10 MINUTES
COOKING TIME: 50 MINUTES

SERVES 6

1 brown onion
4 carrots
4 zucchini (courgettes)
2 celery stalks
¼ cup (5 g) parsley leaves, plus
    extra to garnish
2 tablespoons extra virgin olive oil
two 400 g (14 oz) tins chopped
    tomatoes (or 5–6 fresh
    tomatoes, chopped)
2 tablespoons tomato paste
    (tomato concentrate)
3 garlic cloves
1 tablespoon ground cumin
6 cups (1.5 litres) vegetable stock
400 g (14 oz) tin cannellini beans,
    drained and rinsed
½ teaspoon freshly ground black
    pepper
shaved parmesan cheese, to serve
    (optional)

Tips

- *Make a big batch on the weekend and you'll have healthy meals for the week ahead.*
- *Use whatever vegetables you have and play around with this recipe: it's simply a guide!*
- *The longer the soup cooks for, the better it'll get. My bobba (my Yiddish nonna) used to cook soups for three days before serving! What a marathon. Though that slow-living philosophy is inspiring, I don't have time, so I cut the cooking time. Of course, you can't compare the two, but she used to say, 'done is better than perfect'!*

As I don't have a dishwasher minimal cleaning up is important to me, and this one-tray dish is about as easy as it gets. This may be the perfect meal to have after a busy day because it's so quick and simple and you'll still be able to climb into bed with time to unwind.

Maple soy sriracha one-tray salmon

PREP TIME: 5 MINUTES
COOKING TIME: 15 MINUTES

SERVES: 2

2 pieces of salmon or trout,
  120 g (4¼ oz) each
1 broccoli head, chopped into
  small florets
1 red capsicum (pepper), sliced,
  seeds removed
2 carrots, thinly sliced
cooked brown rice, to serve
1 tablespoon sesame seeds
  (optional), to serve

MARINADE
2 tablespoons soy sauce or tamari
  (gluten-free soy sauce)
1 tablespoon maple syrup
1 tablespoon sriracha (or chilli
  sauce)
2 tablespoons water

Preheat the oven to 200°C (400°F). Line a baking tray with baking paper or foil and arrange the fish and vegetables on it.

Combine the ingredients for the marinade in a small jug and mix well. Pour the marinade over the fish and vegetables on the tray and bake for 15 minutes.

Serve with brown rice, sprinkled with sesame seeds, if using.

Tips

- The combination of maple syrup, soy sauce and sriracha is insanely tasty and is my go-to marinade for lots of barbecued meats and vegetables.
- Sriracha is a popular chilli sauce available from almost all supermarkets; however, you can use any mild chilli-based sauce instead. If you use sweet chilli sauce, leave out the maple syrup.
- I love using precooked serves of brown rice, which are perfect to accompany this meal.
- Use up whatever vegetables you have in this dish, such as asparagus, brussels sprouts, squash, zucchini (courgettes), red cabbage, onion and so on.

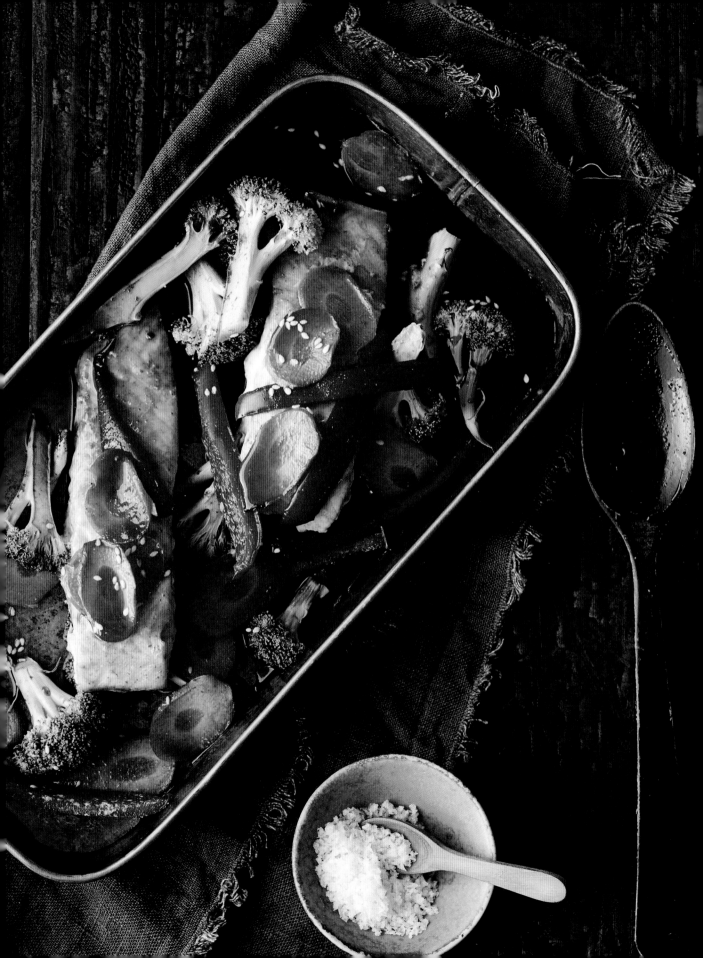

everyday option • dairy free • low gi • high fibre • heart healthy • healthy ageing • diabetes friendly • nut free

Stir-fries are my choice for a quick and nutritious meal that I know my family will eat. This one is simple and tastes as good as it looks. I love to cut the vegies on the diagonal for no other reason than it looks nice!

Green chicken stir-fry

PREP TIME: 10 MINUTES
COOKING TIME: 15 MINUTES

SERVES 4

2 tablespoons extra virgin olive oil
2 teaspoons sesame oil
1 brown onion, sliced
500 g (1 lb 2 oz) lean chicken
    mince
2 garlic cloves, finely chopped
2 long red chilli, sliced
2 baby broccoli (broccolini), sliced
250 g (7 oz) button mushrooms,
    sliced
2 bunches pak choy, sliced
Cooked brown rice, to serve

SAUCE
3 tablespoons soy sauce
2 tablespoons sweet chilli sauce
2 tablespoons oyster sauce
1 tablespoon freshly grated ginger

Combine the ingredients for the sauce in a small bowl and mix well. Set aside.

Heat a wok to medium-high and add the olive and sesame oils and the onion. Cook for 2 minutes. Add the chicken, breaking up lumps. Cook for 4–5 minutes.

Add the garlic, chilli and baby broccoli. Cook for 2 minutes. Add the mushrooms and the sauce and cook for 3 minutes. Add the pak choy and cook for a further 2 minutes.

Serve with brown rice for a delicious and healthy dinner.

Tips

- I love baby broccoli (a mix between broccoli and gai larn, Chinese broccoli). If you can't find it, ordinary broccoli is a wonderful and convenient alternative.
- If you can't find pak choy (Chinese spinach) at your supermarket or Asian grocery store, simply use spinach or swiss chard.
- Use tamari (gluten-free soy sauce) instead of soy sauce if you want to make this gluten free.

My secret weapon for awesome-tasting salad is adding sweet potato crisps in place of croutons. Yes, they're fried and not the healthiest ingredient, but boy, oh boy, it'll make everyone a salad fan. It's not an everyday option but it's the perfect trick when you're asked to bring salad to a party and want to impress.

Hail Caesar salad with creamy avocado dressing

Put the eggs in a small saucepan and cover with water. Bring to a boil, then cook for 6 minutes. Drain and run the eggs under cold water. Peel and cut into quarters.

Put the dressing ingredients into a food processor and blitz until smooth and creamy.

Arrange the salad ingredients in a serving bowl. Drizzle with the dressing and top with the crisps (if using) just before serving.

PREP TIME: 10 MINUTES
COOKING TIME: 10 MINUTES

SERVES 4

4 eggs
4 baby cos lettuce, roughly chopped
½ small red onion, sliced
1 cup (150 g) cherry tomatoes, sliced
¼ cup (25 g) parmesan cheese, shaved
1 small packet (85 g) sweet potato crisps (optional), to serve

AVOCADO DRESSING

1 ripe avocado
2 garlic cloves
Juice of 1 lime and 1 lemon (or 1½ lemons)
3 tablespoons extra virgin olive oil
½ teaspoon salt
½ cup (125 ml) water
½ cup mint or parsley, coarsely chopped (optional)

Tips

- *Be sure to put the crisps on only at the last minute, to keep them, well... crisp!*
- *Thanks to the citrus, the avocado dressing will keep for a couple of weeks in your fridge in an airtight container. It's great with loads of other salads, especially those such as coleslaw that need a creamy dressing.*
- *You can add chicken to this salad or use kale instead of cos lettuce.*
- *Leave out the parmesan cheese to make it dairy free.*

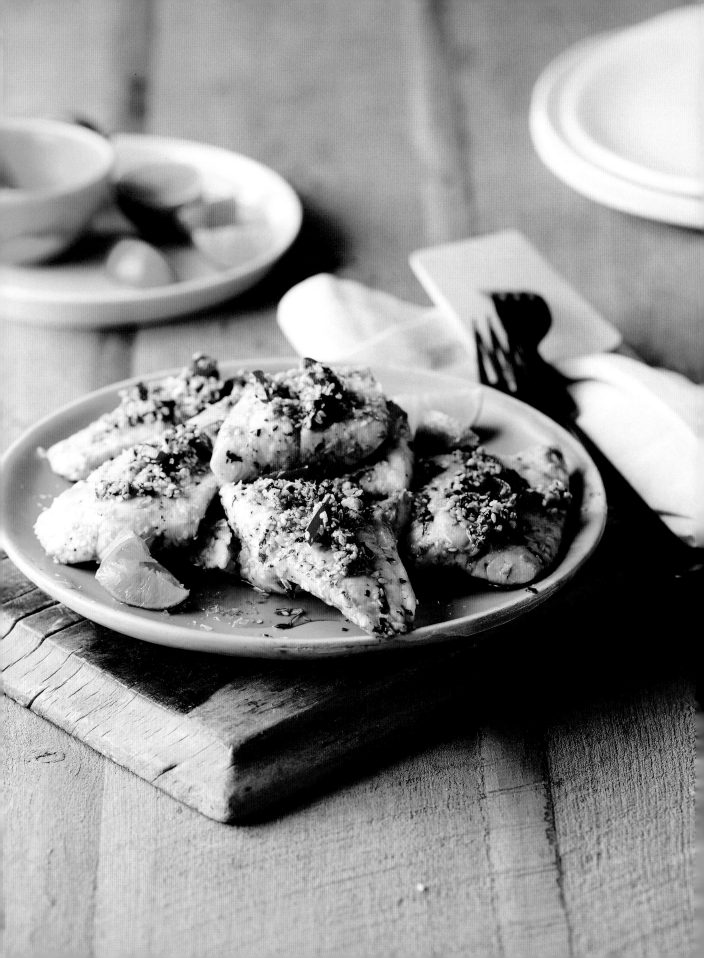

After a weekend of big eating, some delicious fish served with salad tends to be my preference come Monday. White fish is super-easy to cook, but adding a delicious marinade or crust can take it to the next level.

Sesame-crusted fish

Combine all of the ingredients except the fish and extra sesame seeds in a small bowl. Add the fish and coat well.

Heat a medium frying pan over medium-high heat. Cook the fish fillets for 3 minutes on each side.

Sprinkle with the toasted sesame seeds and serve with lime wedges.

PREP TIME: 5 MINUTES
COOKING TIME: 6 MINUTES

SERVES 2

1 tablespoon extra virgin olive oil
1 teaspoon sesame oil
1 cm (⅜ inch) piece ginger, grated
¼ cup (15 g) chopped coriander (cilantro) leaves
1 chilli, sliced
1 tablespoon lime juice
½ teaspoon mixed pepper and salt
1 tablespoon sesame seeds, plus extra, toasted, to serve
2 firm white-fleshed fish fillets, about 100 g (3½ oz) each
lime wedges, to serve

Tips

- Double or triple this recipe if you're cooking for a family or a group of friends, or so you have plenty of leftovers.
- I love to serve this with the Eat the rainbow grated salad (see page 206) and brown rice or throw together some fish tacos by stuffing tortillas with sliced red cabbage and avocado and topping with hot sauce.
- Don't like coriander (cilantro)? Skip it or use parsley leaves instead.

This dish takes 10 minutes to throw together, then you can simply set and forget. By dinner time, you'll have a very yummy, balanced meal. When it comes time to serve, break apart the chicken with a fork and you'll get more mileage from less meat.

Quinoa burrito bowl in the slow cooker

PREP TIME: 10 MINUTES

COOKING TIME: 4–6 HOURS IN A SLOW COOKER

SERVES 4–5

1 cup (200 g) quinoa, rinsed

400 g (14 oz) tin sweet corn, drained

400 g (14 oz) tin black beans, drained

2 red chillies, chopped (or 1 tablespoon chilli flakes)

2 garlic cloves

two 400 g (14 oz) tins crushed tomatoes

1 tablespoon sweet paprika

2 teaspoons ground cumin

2 teaspoons ground turmeric

1 brown onion, chopped

1 red capsicum (pepper), seeds removed, chopped

4 chicken thighs, chopped into 2.5 cm (1 inch) pieces

2 cups (500 ml) vegetable stock

Coriander (cilantro) or parsley leaves and lime wedges, to serve

Avocado slices and extra sliced chilli, to serve (optional)

Combine all of the ingredients in a slow cooker and stir well. Set the slow cooker to high and cook for 4–6 hours.

Scatter with coriander or parsley leaves and squeeze lime juice over. Serve with sliced avocado and extra sliced chilli, if desired.

Tips

- *If you're vegan, vegetarian or keen for a meat-free meal, simply skip the chicken!*
- *If you want more heat, enjoy this with your favourite hot sauce.*
- *Serve with wholegrain corn chips and hot sauce for a seriously good feed.*

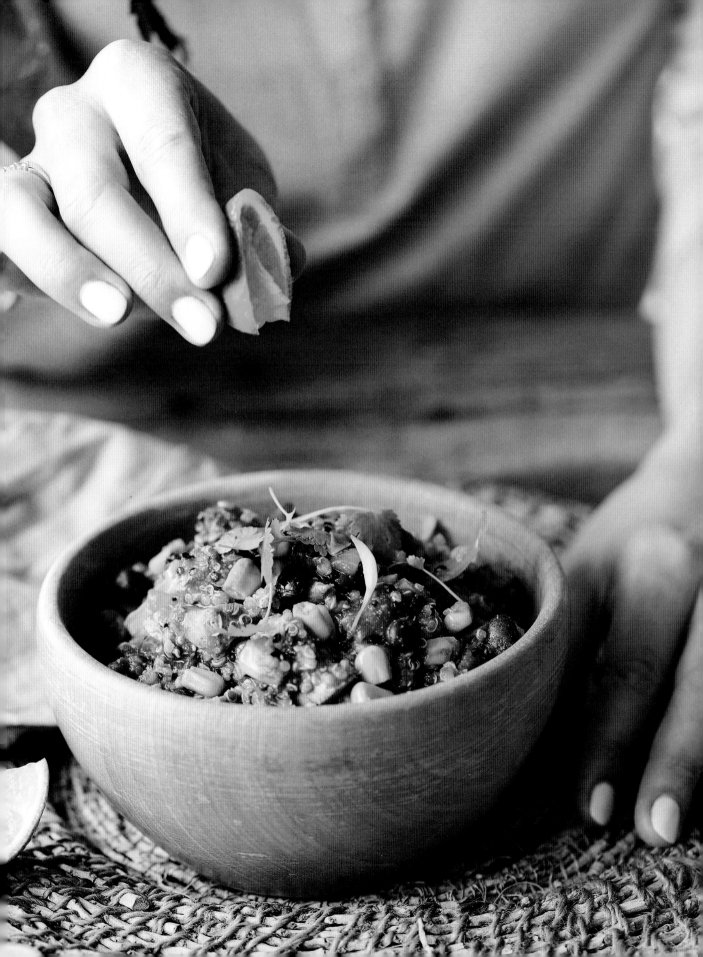

Don't have time to make dinner? Don't stress. This dish is a real life-saver when you haven't got time for meal prep. Healthy eating has to be convenient and easy.

Cheater's chicken slaw

PREP TIME: 10 MINUTES

SERVES 4

1 roast chicken, skin and bones removed, meat shredded
500 g (1 lb 2 oz) kaleslaw or coleslaw mix (leave out the dressing)
½ cup (15 g) coriander (cilantro) or mint leaves
1 red chilli, chopped
½ cup spring onion (scallions) or red onion, finely chopped
1 teaspoon sesame seeds, to serve
¼ cup (35 g) peanuts, to serve (optional)

DRESSING
3 tablespoons extra virgin olive oil
2 tablespoons soy sauce
½ teaspoon sesame oil
2 tablespoons lime juice
1 teaspoon freshly grated ginger
1 garlic clove, finely chopped
1 teaspoon honey

Combine all of the dressing ingredients in a small bowl or jug and mix well.

Toss the chicken, kaleslaw mix, coriander or mint, chilli, spring onion and sesame seeds together in a bowl.

Pour the dressing over and toss to coat. Top with sesame seeds and peanuts (if using).

Tips

- Most supermarkets serve a wonderful premixed 'coleslaw' with shredded carrots, cabbage and sometimes kale or herbs. I love these mixes because they save me time and cleaning up. I also love buying a roasted free-range chicken from the supermarket because I like to make things easy for myself.
- The magic of this recipe is in the dressing, which is all you need to make a good meal taste great. Use mint instead if you don't love coriander (cilantro).
- Use tamari (gluten-free soy sauce) if you are sensitive to gluten.
- Skip the peanuts if you are allergic.

Fish and chips is a classic, and no-one can deny it. So let's not deny ourselves this delicious food, by simply swapping it for a healthier version like this seedy crumbed fish.

Seedy crumbed fish

Put the almonds, pepitas and sunflower seeds, parmesan and garlic into a food processor (or use a mortar and pestle) and process until you have coarse crumbs.

Spray the fish with olive oil and coat with the crumb mixture. Season with salt and pepper.

Heat a nonstick frying pan over medium-high heat and fry the fish for 3 minutes on each side until crumbs are golden brown.

PREP TIME: 5 MINUTES
COOKING TIME: 6 MINUTES

SERVES 2

¼ cup (40 g) roasted almonds
2 tablespoons pepitas (pumpkin seeds)
2 tablespoons sunflower seeds
2 tablespoons finely grated parmesan cheese
1 garlic clove, finely chopped (or ½ teaspoon garlic powder)
2 boneless white fish fillets, such as ocean perch or snapper, about 150 g (5½ oz) each
olive oil spray

Tips

- If I've got time, I'll slice up some sweet potato (the thinner, the better), toss with salt, pepper and extra virgin olive oil and bake in the oven for 30 minutes.
- Don't love fish? Use this recipe with chicken instead. Pan-fry for 10 minutes or until cooked to make healthy chicken nuggets.
- You can bake the fish in the oven at 200°C (400°F) for 10 minutes.

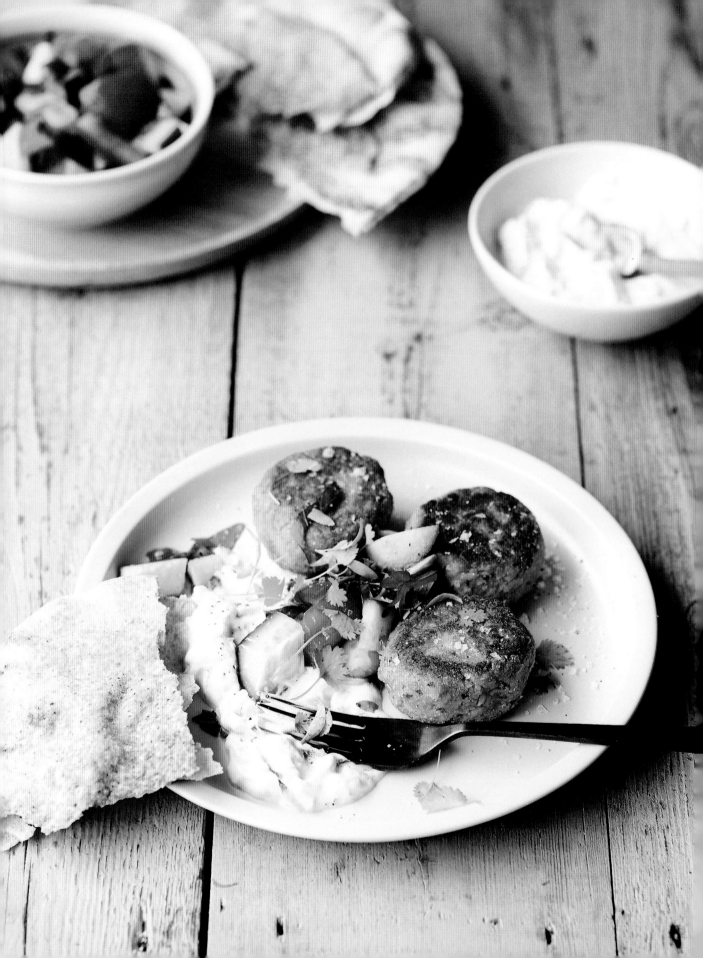

The falafel are super moist so you can eat them the next day. My favourite bit is that they are so ridiculously simple to make. I love having baked pumpkin in my fridge (it's one of my favourite vegies) and once a week I'll do the Life-saving baked rainbow vegies on page 200 as meal prep, then use some of the pumpkin for this recipe.

Pumpkin falafel

Put all of the ingredients, except for the olive oil, into a food processor and blitz for 30 seconds or until smooth. Roll into balls, then press down to flatten slightly.

Heat the olive oil in a large frying pan over medium–high heat. Add the falafel balls and cook for 2 minutes on each side. Drain on paper towel.

PREP: 5 MINUTES
COOKING TIME: 4 MINUTES

SERVES: 4 (MAKES AROUND 20)

1 cup cooked peeled kent pumpkin (squash)
two 400 g (14 oz) tins chickpeas (garbanzo beans), drained and rinsed
2 teaspoons ground cumin
2 garlic cloves
½ cup (70 g) wholemeal plain flour
½ cup (10 g) parsley leaves
2 tablespoons extra virgin olive oil, for cooking

Tips

- If you haven't any baked pumpkin on hand, peel 400–500 g (14 oz–1 lb 2 oz) of pumpkin and bake it at 200°C (400°F) for 45 minutes or until soft.
- Enjoy the falafel balls with a salad or serve with Cheeky tzatziki (see page 210), wholemeal pita bread and Quinoa pomegranate tabouleh (see page 192).
- Use gluten-free flour if you're sensitive.

Tacos can be fresh, tasty and really nutritious. They're especially great for midweek family meals because you can serve them buffet style, so everyone can create combinations they love.

Twenty-minute tacos

PREP TIME: 10 MINUTES

COOKING TIME: 10 MINUTES

SERVES 4–6

400 g (14 oz) boneless, skinless
  chicken thighs

2½ cups (300 g) cherry tomatoes,
  quartered

¼ red onion, chopped

½ Lebanese cucumber, chopped

8–12 wholegrain tortillas or
  small wraps

2 baby cos or ½ iceberg lettuce

1 avocado

1 lime, cut into wedges

Coriander (cilantro) or mint leaves,
  to serve (optional)

MARINADE

2 tablespoons soy sauce

1 tablespoon sweet chilli sauce

1 teaspoon sesame oil

Combine the ingredients for the marinade in a medium bowl. Cut the chicken into small pieces and toss with the marinade in the bowl.

Heat a barbecue or chargrill pan to medium-high heat. Cook the chicken for 5 minutes on each side or until cooked through.

Combine the tomato, onion and cucumber in a bowl to make a fresh salsa and season with salt and pepper.

Set out the taco ingredients separately in buffet style: wholegrain tortillas, lettuce leaves, fresh salsa, avocado, chicken, lime wedges and coriander (if using).

Tips

- You can replace the chicken with the Seedy crumbed fish (see page 185) or Terrifically tasty teriyaki salmon (see page 171) to make fish tacos.
- Pretty much any sliced veg is a hit in a taco, so play around with different combinations; just make sure they're sliced thinly.
- If you've got five extra minutes, whip up the Holy moly guacamole on page 208 and use it in place of the avocado.
- Use gluten-free tortillas and tamari (gluten-free soy sauce) if you are sensitive.

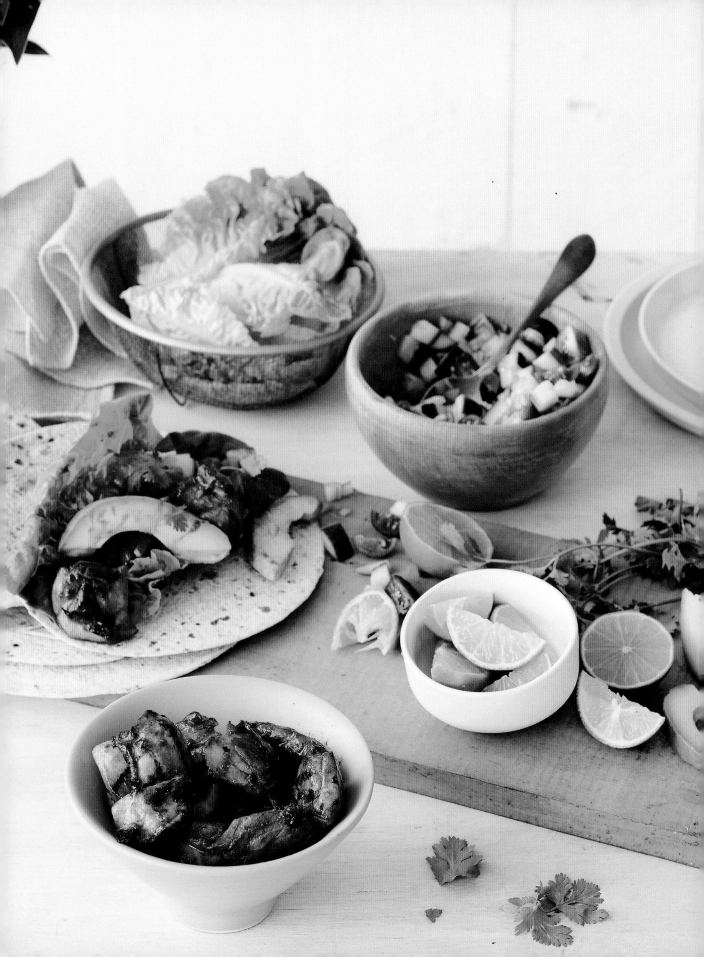

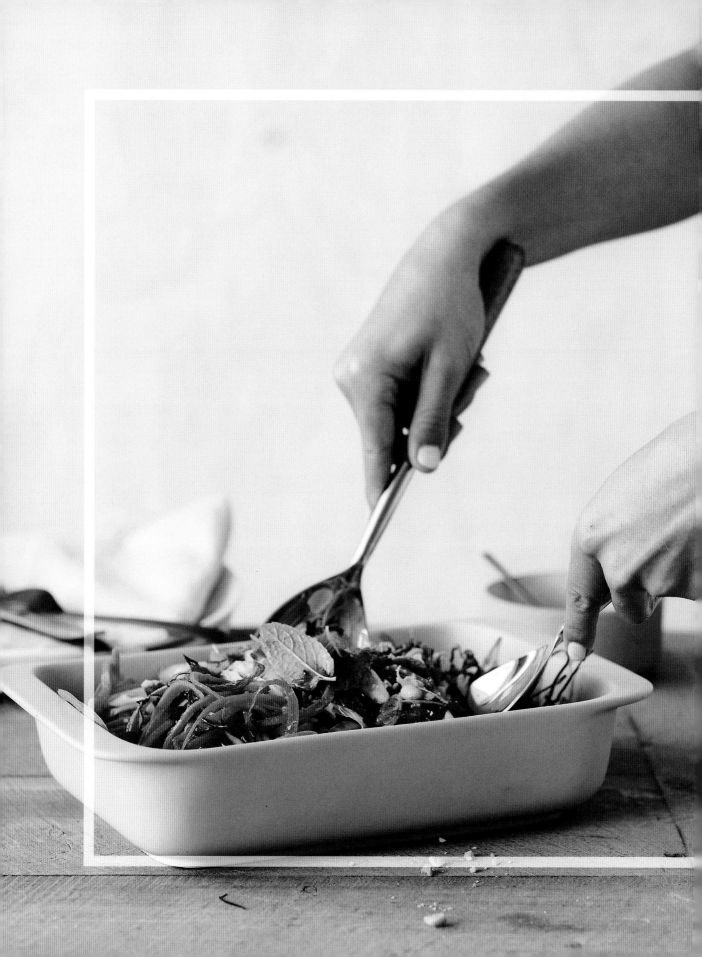

salads, vegies, dips and sauces

This recipe is ideal for meal prep in advance (or perfect for camping) because it keeps well in an airtight container. I serve this with grilled fish, Pumpkin falafel (see page 187) or add it to Mumma's meatballs (see page 170).

Quinoa pomegranate tabouleh

PREP TIME: 10 MINUTES
COOKING TIME: 20 MINUTES

SERVES 6

1 cup (200 g) quinoa (or 2 cups
    cooked quinoa)
2–3 large tomatoes, finely
    chopped
1 cup (20 g) parsley leaves,
    finely chopped
4 spring onions (scallions),
    finely chopped
Juice of 1 lemon
1 pomegranate (see tips for
    collecting seeds)
¼ teaspoon salt

Cook quinoa as per instructions in 4 cups boiling water for 20 minutes or until soft but still chewy. Drain and set aside to cool.

Meanwhile, put the chopped tomato into a sieve to drain slightly.

Combine all of the ingredients in a salad bowl, toss well and serve.

Tips

- If you can't find pomegranate or it isn't in season, use currants instead or simply leave out the fruit. It's still going to be an incredibly tasty and healthy salad.
- Deseeding a pomegranate can be chore. To make it less painful (and messy), scoop the seeds into a bowl and then fill the bowl with water. The bitter white pith will float to the top, making it easy to remove. Drain well, and the seeds are ready to use.

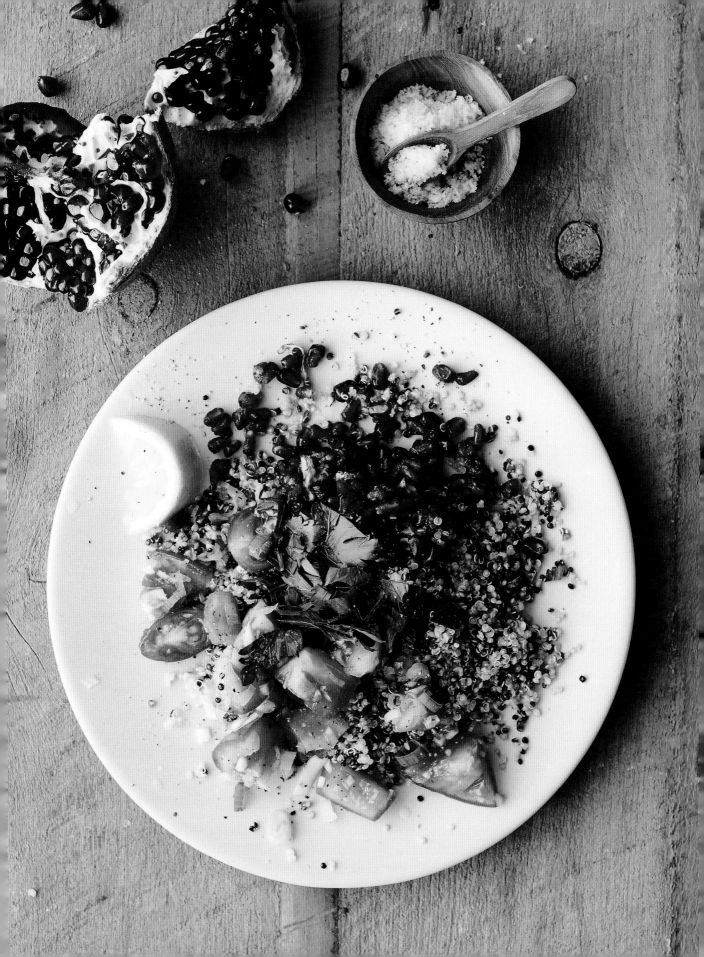

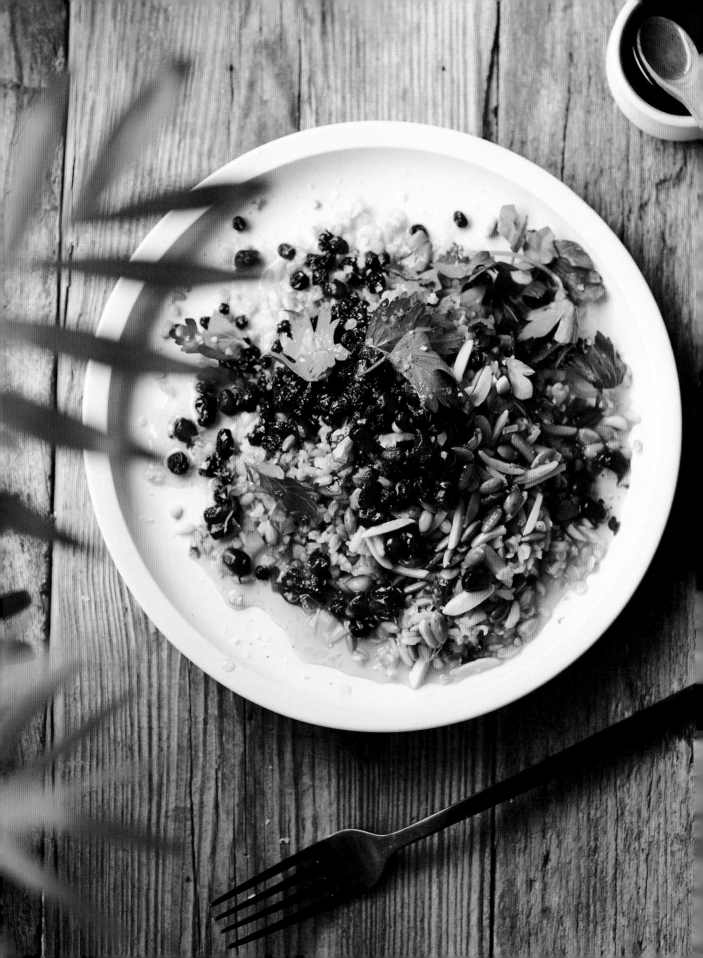

Freekeh is my favourite wholegrain. It used to be really hard to find, but it's becoming more popular and is available from most large supermarkets and health-food shops.

Freeken' good freekeh salad

Preheat the oven to 180°C (350°F).

Put the freekeh in a saucepan with 6 cups (1.5 litres) of cold water and bring to the boil over high heat. Cover the pan with a lid and reduce the heat to simmer for 20 minutes or until cooked.

Meanwhile, put the currants in a small bowl with 1 cup (250 ml) cold water to soak.

Spread the almonds, pepitas and pine nuts on a baking tray lined with baking paper. Roast for 2–3 minutes or until golden brown. Watch the seeds and nuts VERY closely so you don't burn them.

Drain the freekeh well and put it in a large salad bowl. Toss with the onion, pomegranate seeds, half the parsley, the toasted nuts and seeds and the drained currants. To serve, toss with the dressing and remaining parsley.

PREP TIME: 10 MINUTES
COOKING TIME: 20 MINUTES

SERVES 6

2 cups (400 g) cracked freekeh
1 cup (140 g) dried currants
½ cup (65 g) slivered almonds
½ cup (75 g) pepitas (pumpkin
   seeds)
½ cup (80 g) pine nuts or
   sunflower seeds
1 small red onion, finely chopped
Seeds from ½ pomegranate
1 cup (20 g) parsley leaves,
   coarsely chopped

HONEY LIME DRESSING
½ cup (125 ml) extra virgin olive oil
1 tablespoon of honey
juice of 2 limes
1 teaspoon salt

Tips

- Make this salad at the start of a busy week and it'll keep really well in the fridge in an airtight container.
- Use quinoa instead of freekeh to make this recipe gluten free.
- Use either cracked or uncracked freekeh for this recipe. It's all good. Simply follow the cooking instructions on the back of the packet for uncracked freekeh.
- Use maple syrup instead of honey to make this recipe vegan.

When I can't be bothered cooking, this kind of thing happens: I raid the pantry and fridge and grab whatever I can find. I always have beans on hand, as well as tins of tuna, olives and seeds. Then I add as much veg as possible and my lunch is ready. In five minutes, I have a balanced Mediterranean feast, which just goes to show that it doesn't take long to create healthy, yummy meals.

Mediterranean lunch bowl

PREP TIME: 5 MINUTES

SERVES: 1

200 g (7 oz) tinned chickpeas
    (garbanzo beans)
1 cup (40 g) salad leaves
100 g (3½ oz) tinned tuna, drained
½ Lebanese (short) cucumber,
    chopped
1 tomato, chopped
2 tablespoons olives, pitted
1 tablespoon toasted seeds, such
    as sunflower seeds, pepitas
    (pumpkin seeds), linseeds
    (flaxseeds)
1 teaspoon balsamic glaze

Arrange all ingredients in a medium bowl and drizzle with the balsamic glaze.

Tip

- *Balsamic glaze is a reduced mixture of balsamic vinegar and sugar syrup and is available from supermarkets. Alternatively, use balsamic vinegar and extra virgin olive oil as a great salad dressing.*

Depending on the season, I've got you covered with my loaded Greek salad, which is delicious done either way. In spring and summer, use olives. Enjoy it with pomegranate seeds during the cooler months.

Loaded Greek salad, two ways

Combine the ingredients for the dressing in a small bowl or jug.

Put all of the salad ingredients except the feta and olive oil into a salad bowl. Serve the feta as a wedge in the middle of the bowl, then drizzle lightly with extra virgin olive oil.

Serve with the dressing.

Tips

- *Add some protein, such as a couple of boiled eggs or a tin of tuna, for a complete meal.*
- *This is a fantastic lunch to take to work.*
- *Serve it with Mumma's meatballs (see page 170) or the Sesame-crusted fish (see page 181).*
- *Leave out the feta to make this recipe dairy free. Swap the honey for maple syrup to make it vegan.*

PREP TIME: 10 MINUTES

SERVES 4

½ red onion, sliced
400 g (14 oz) tin of chickpeas (garbanzo beans), drained and rinsed
1 Lebanese cucumber, chopped
1 large ripe tomato, chopped
¼ cup (5 g) mint leaves
1 teaspoon finely grated lemon zest
½ cup (75 g) pitted kalamata olives, chopped (spring and summer)
Seeds from ½ pomegranate (autumn and winter)
100 g (3½ oz) feta cheese
olive oil, to serve

DRESSING
3 tablespoons lemon juice
6 tablespoons extra virgin olive oil
1 tablespoon honey
1 garlic clove, finely chopped

One tray of baked goodness coming right up! Enjoy this as a baked dish on its own or layer it on a bed of fresh rocket (arugula) or baby spinach for a delicious salad.

Baked pumpkin with feta

PREP TIME: 10 MINUTES
COOKING TIME: 1 HOUR 10 MINUTES

SERVES 6

2 red onions
½ small kent pumpkin (squash), skin on, about 1 kg (2 lb 4 oz)
2 tablespoons balsamic vinegar
2 tablespoons extra virgin olive oil
⅓ cup (50 g) pine nuts
⅓ cup (50 g) crumbled Danish feta cheese
¼ cup (15 g) chopped parsley

Preheat the oven to 200°C (400°F). Line a baking tray with baking paper.

Slice each onion into six wedges. Chop the pumpkin in wedges about the same thickness as the onion. Keep the skin on!

Spread the wedges of onion and pumpkin on the prepared tray and drizzle with the balsamic vinegar and olive oil. Bake for 1 hour or until caramelised. Add the pine nuts and cook for a further 10 minutes.

Serve with crumbled feta and parsley.

Tips

- This recipe is best with kent pumpkin (squash), which has green and cream speckled skin. It caramelises and goes so incredibly gooey. You're gonna love this!
- You can eat the skin of the pumpkin. It's delicious and high in fibre!
- Try mint instead of parsley and chopped almonds or pepitas (pumpkin seeds) instead of pine nuts.

salads, vegies, dips and sauces

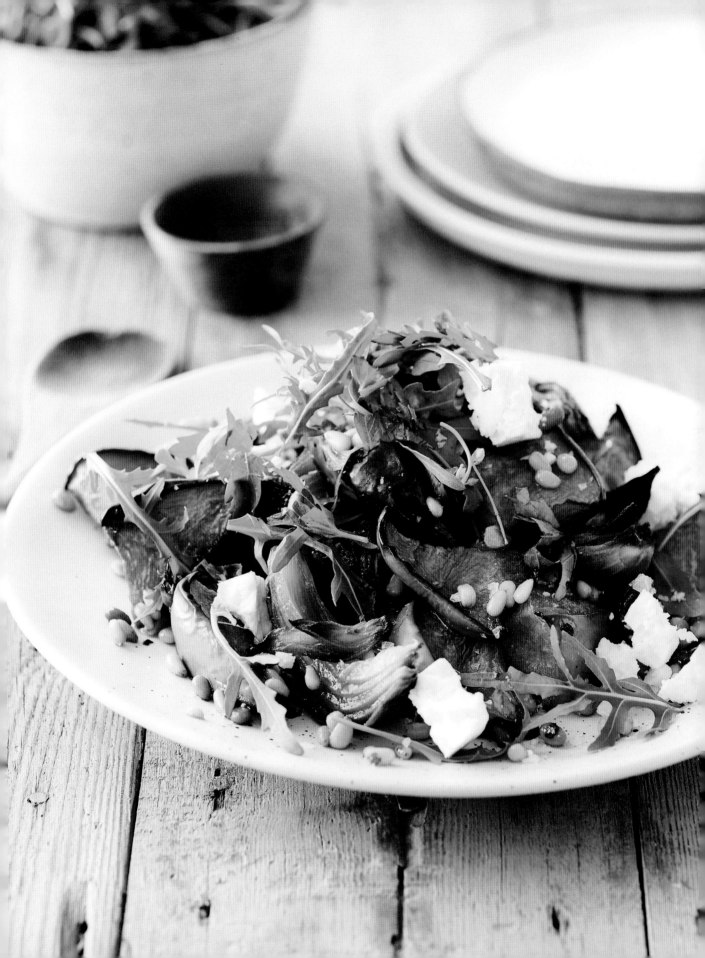

Having loads of baked vegetables in the fridge is kinda lifesaving. Suddenly, you'll find healthy eating is much easier because the hard work has already been done. Meal prep can be overwhelming, so I prioritise this one recipe. Store the vegies in the fridge in airtight containers.

Lifesaving baked rainbow vegetables

PREP TIME: 15 MINUTES

COOKING TIME: 1 HOUR

2 capsicum (peppers), 1 red
    and 1 yellow, seeds removed,
    chopped
500 g (1 lb 2 oz) pumpkin (squash),
    peeled and chopped
1 red onion, cut into wedges
1 broccoli, cut into florets
4 carrots, sliced
2 teaspoons paprika
2 teaspoons turmeric
1 teaspoon salt
3 tablespoons extra virgin olive oil

SEASONAL VARIATIONS

Red: cherry tomatoes
Yellow: baby squash, yellow
    tomatoes, yellow beetroot
Orange: sweet potato, orange
    tomatoes
Green: zucchini (courgettes),
    brussels sprouts, green
    capsicum (peppers), asparagus,
    green beans
Purple: beetroot, purple yams,
    eggplant (aubergine)

Preheat the oven to 200°C (400°F). Line 2 baking trays with baking paper and spread the vegetables on them (be sure not to crowd the veg). Sprinkle with the spices, salt and half the olive oil then toss the vegetables. Cook for 45 minutes to 1 hour.

Remove from oven and toss with the remaining oil. Season with salt.

Tips

- *You can have a pumpkin and beetroot salad one day, and serve broccoli and sweet potato with your grilled fish on another day.*
- *I also love to use Italian spice mix or roast vegetable spice mix instead of the paprika and turmeric because it's so easy. Really, almost any spices will work here!*
- *If you bake and store the vegetables separately, you'll have a little more flexibility with how you use them during the week.*

Quick and easy greens? These are so good, they'll get snatched up before you even look around. I serve them in the frying pan to save washing up.

Chilli garlic snow peas

Heat the olive and sesame oils in a frying pan over high heat. Add the snow peas, chilli and garlic and a pinch of salt.

Sauté for 3 minutes. Sprinkle with sesame seeds and squeeze lemon juice over.

PREP TIME: 5 MINUTES
COOKING TIME: 3 MINUTES

SERVES 2

1 teaspoon extra virgin olive oil
1 teaspoon sesame oil
250 g (9 oz) snow peas, trimmed
1 chilli, finely chopped, or
¼ teaspoon chilli flakes
1 garlic clove, finely chopped
1–2 teaspoons of sesame seeds,
to serve
Lemon wedges, to serve

Tips

- Top with toasted slivered almonds instead of the sesame seeds.
- This would be great served with grilled fish and wholegrains.

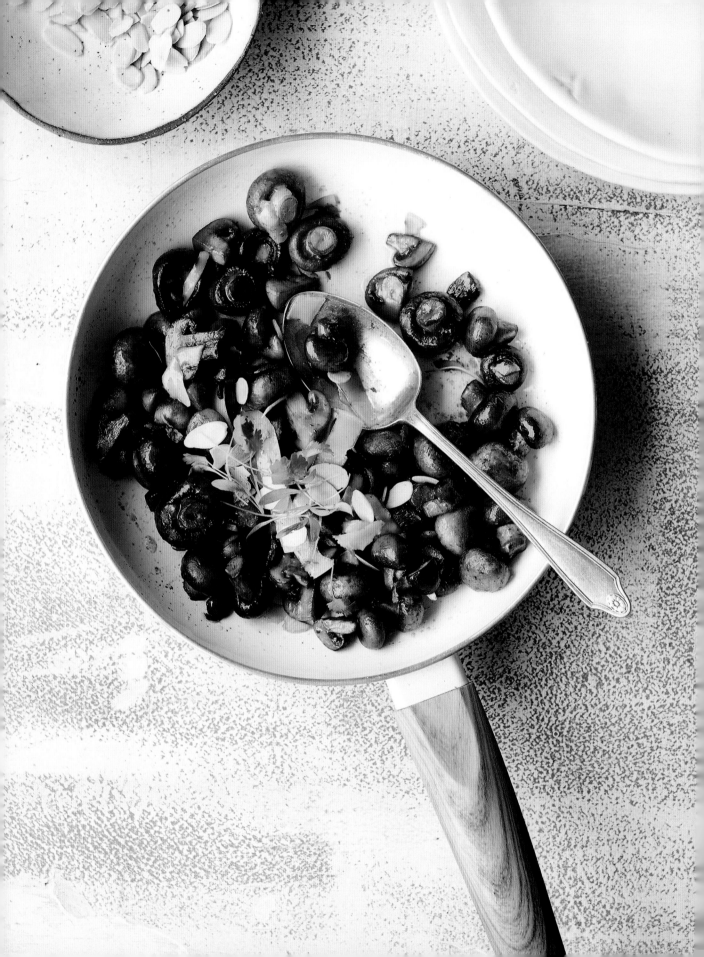

I believe with all my heart that vegetables should be the star attraction on any plate, cooked with delicious flavours and ingredients. Healthy food must contain nutrients, but also needs to feed the soul, don't you think? These garlicky parmesan mushrooms do just that. This is comfort food that's also good for you.

Garlicky parmesan mushrooms

Heat a large frying pan over medium-high heat. Toast the almonds for 1–2 minutes, tossing to prevent them from burning. Remove from the pan and set aside.

Add the olive oil to the frying pan. When it's hot, add the mushrooms and cook for 3 minutes, tossing once or twice. Add the garlic, salt and parmesan and cook for 1 minute more, until the cheese has melted.

Serve scattered with the parsley and toasted almonds.

PREP TIME: 2 MINUTES
COOKING TIME: 7 MINUTES

SERVES 4

2 tablespoons flaked almonds

1 tablespoon extra virgin olive oil

6 cups button mushrooms, quartered

2–3 garlic cloves, finely chopped

½ teaspoon salt

3 tablespoons finely grated parmesan cheese

⅓ cup (20 g) chopped parsley

Tip

- *Mushrooms are an incredible vegetable that don't get enough credit. Leave 100 g (3½ oz) in the sun for an hour and they'll give you 100 per cent of your vitamin D needs for the day. A lack of vitamin D is linked with seasonal depression, so this simple hack is handy during winter, when the sun doesn't shine often.*

Like maple-glazed bacon, this is similarly moreish. This recipe goes perfectly
with oily fish, such as salmon or trout, and red meat.

Maple-chilli sauté greens

PREP TIME: 5 MINUTES
COOKING TIME: 10 MINUTES

SERVES 4

¼ cup (25 g) flaked almonds
1 tablespoon extra virgin olive oil
16 asparagus spears
1 chilli, chopped, or 1 teaspoon
   chilli flakes
¼ teaspoon salt
1 tablespoon maple syrup

Heat a frying pan over medium heat and toast the
almonds for 5 minutes or until golden brown. Remove
from the pan and set aside.

Add the olive oil to the frying pan. When the oil is hot,
add the asparagus to the pan with the chilli, salt and
maple syrup. Cover with a lid and cook for 5 minutes,
tossing occasionally.

Serve topped with the toasted almonds.

Tips

- Use pure maple syrup, not maple-flavoured
  syrup, which is more processed.
- To test if the oil in the pan is hot enough,
  flick a few drops of water into the pan with
  your fingertips. When it sizzles, it's ready!
- This recipe is also great with baby broccoli
  (broccolini), broccoli florets and Asian greens.

A truly delectable salad dressing is best when it has:
• Something fatty: extra virgin olive oil, avocado, tahini, sesame oil, yoghurt
• Something acid: vinegar, cider, lime or lemon juice
• Something salty: soy sauce, tamari (gluten-free soy sauce), feta cheese, nuts
• Something sweet: honey, maple syrup, raw sugar, fresh fruit

Salad dressings

Tahini dressing

A fabulous dressing to toss through coleslaw in place of a mayonnaise-based option. I also love this dressing drizzled on roasted vegetables.

SERVES 6

2 tablespoons tahini
2 tablespoons extra virgin olive oil
2 tablespoons lime or lemon juice
1 garlic clove, crushed
¼ teaspoon sea salt
1–2 tablespoons warm water (add until runny)

Poke bowl dressing

Pour this dressing over Eat the rainbow grated salad (see page 206) and serve with 100 g (3½ oz) of sliced raw sashimi-grade salmon for a delicious poke bowl.

SERVES 1–2

3 tablespoons soy sauce or tamari (gluten-free soy sauce)
2 tablespoons lime juice
½ teaspoon sesame oil
1½ teaspoons grated fresh ginger
1 teaspoon of sesame seeds

Basic balsamic dressing

The perfect dressing to go with pretty much any salad. I always make a big batch and keep a jar of this dressing handy.

SERVES 8–10

½ cup (125 ml) extra virgin olive oil
3 tablespoons white wine vinegar
3 tablespoons balsamic vinegar
1 heaped teaspoon dijon mustard

Tip

• *For the perfect balance, add fat and acid at a 2:1 ratio. For example, ½ cup (125 ml) of oil and ¼ cup (60 ml) of apple cider vinegar. Then add sweetness (1 tablespoon of honey), a pinch of salt and some fresh herbs. Viola! A delicious salad dressing is born.*

You'll get a golden glow at the end of this rainbow salad from all the beautiful nutrients. Luckily, this salad tastes as good as it looks. Best bit? It's equally great for meal prep or entertaining.

Eat the rainbow grated salad

PREP TIME: 15 MINUTES

SERVES 8

½ purple cabbage, sliced

2 carrots, spiralised or very thinly sliced

1 red capsicum (pepper), deseeded and thinly sliced

4 spring onions (scallions), sliced

1 cup (20 g) mint leaves

2 avocados, sliced

¼ cup (35 g) peanuts, toasted and crushed

ZESTY DRESSING

3 tablespoons extra virgin olive oil

Juice of 1 lemon

3 tablespoons soy sauce

3 tablespoons sweet chilli sauce

2 teaspoons sesame oil

Combine the cabbage, carrot, capsicum, spring onion and mint in a large bowl. Combine the dressing ingredients in a small bowl and mix well. Toss the dressing through the salad. Top with avocado and serve with toasted peanuts.

Tips

- *Use a v-slicer or mandolin (available from most homewares shops) to thinly slice the cabbage and save a stack of time. Just be really careful as the blade is super sharp!*
- *If you keep the dressing, avocado and nuts separate to add just before serving, this salad will last in your fridge for the best part of a week.*
- *You can also slice in beetroot (beets), kale and yellow capsicum or toss in cherry tomatoes, corn kernels or pomegranate seeds for even more beautiful colours.*
- *Use tamari (gluten-free soy sauce) if you are sensitive to gluten.*

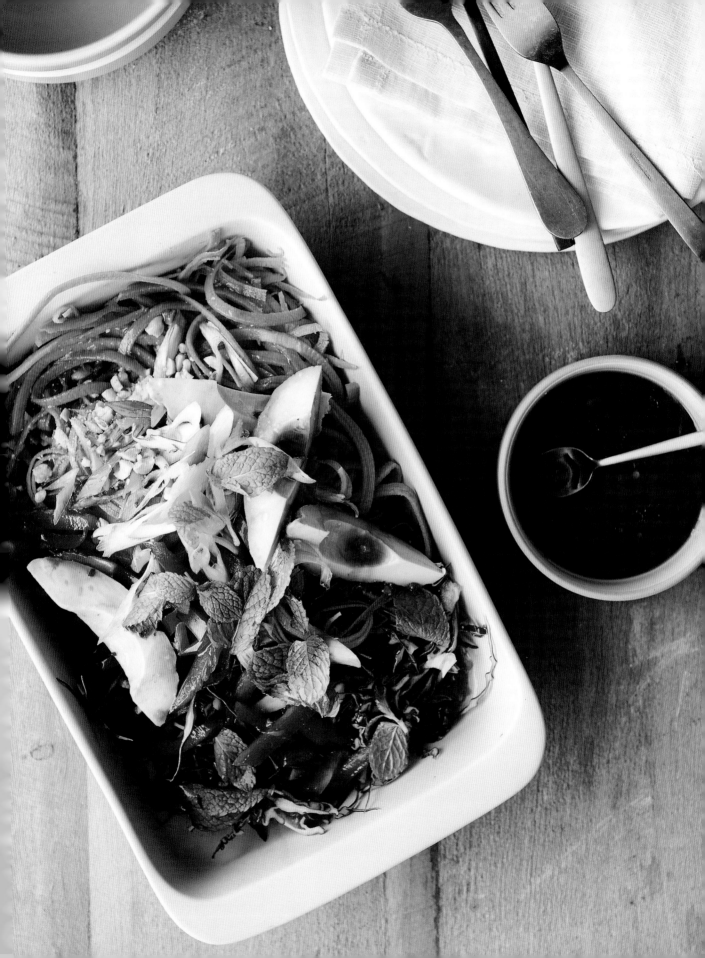

The difference between good guacamole and great guacamole is a few simple ingredients. When you need a nutritious snack, guacamole is always a fantastic option thanks to those heart-loving 'healthy' fats. Serve with chopped vegetables, wholegrain crackers or grainy toast.

Holy moly chunky guacamole!

PREP TIME: 5 MINUTES

SERVES 4

2 small avocados (or 1 large)
1 tomato, finely chopped
¼ red onion, finely chopped
1 garlic clove, crushed
2 tablespoons lemon juice
¼ teaspoon salt
½ teaspoon chilli flakes (optional)
1 tablespoon chopped coriander
   (cilantro) leaves (optional)
40 g (1½ oz) feta cheese (optional)

Coarsely smash the avocado flesh in a small bowl. Add the remaining ingredients and mix through. Taste as you go to get the right combination of flavours.

Tips

- *Guacamole is an awesome accompaniment to main meals: add it to salads as a dressing or dollop on top of cooked meat.*
- *I love to spread guacamole on sandwiches and serve in tacos or wraps.*
- *Leave out the feta to make this dairy free and vegan.*

Steamed, barbecued and grilled vegies alike will love being paired with this peanut sauce. I really do think it is great over any vegetable, but don't just take my word for it: try for yourself!

Pretty perfect peanut sauce

Combine all of the ingredients, stir to mix well and serve on top of your favourite greens.

PREP TIME: 5 MINUTES

SERVES 6

½ cup (140 g) smooth 100%
  peanut butter
1 tablespoon lime juice or
  3 tablespoons rice wine vinegar
3 tablespoons warm water
2 tablespoons soy sauce or tamari
  (gluten-free soy sauce)
1 tablespoon honey or maple syrup
1 garlic clove, crushed
½ teaspoon chilli flakes (optional)

Tips

- *Drizzle over grilled baby broccoli (broccolini), broccoli or asparagus and top with some crushed nuts for a super-delicious side dish, ideal for serving at your next dinner party.*
- *Stir-fry some Asian greens and toss with this dressing.*

Tzatziki is a classic condiment that I love serving with meat, prawns, wraps and salads. It's a killer way to smuggle in another serve of yoghurt (hello probiotics for a healthy gut) and add flavour. If I am serving something heavy or spicy, I'll often whip up a batch of this Cheeky tzatziki because it balances out the flavours perfectly.

Cheeky tzatziki

PREP TIME: 3 MINUTES

SERVES 4

1 cup (260 g) plain Greek-style
    yoghurt
Juice of ½ lime
2 garlic cloves, finely chopped
¼ cup (5 g) parsley leaves,
    chopped

Combine all of the ingredients in a small mixing bowl. Season with salt to taste.

Tip

- *Try Cheeky tzatziki with Mumma's meatballs (see page 170), Pumpkin falafel (see page 187) and the Freeken' good freekeh salad (see page 195).*

everyday option · gluten free · dairy free · vegan · heart healthy · healthy ageing
diabetes friendly · nut free

My husband Les makes this seriously good spicy tomato sauce. Ready-made tomato sauce (or ketchup) is tasty but this is so much more delicious, plus you'll skip all the added sugar and pack a whole lot more flavour and nutrients into your dishes. You'll love the slightly spicy, smokey and sweet flavours in this recipe.

Les's spicy tomato sauce

Blitz the onion, garlic and chilli in a food processor until finely chopped.

Heat the olive oil in a saucepan over medium heat. Add the contents of the food processor and sauté for 3–5 minutes until golden.

Add the sugar, allspice and paprika, stirring occasionally for about 3 minutes until the sugar melts. Add the vinegar, passata and tomato paste and cook for 15–20 minutes until the sauce has thickened.

Transfer to a sterilised jar with an airtight lid. Store for at least 2–3 weeks in the fridge (if it lasts that long).

PREP TIME: 5 MINUTES
COOKING TIME: 25 MINUTES

SERVES 10

1 brown onion
2 garlic cloves
1 long chilli (red or green)
1 tablespoon extra virgin olive oil
3 tablespoons brown sugar
¼ teaspoon ground allspice
½ teaspoon ground smoked paprika
⅓ cup (80 ml) white vinegar
1 cup (125 ml) passata
2 tablespoons tomato paste (concentrated purée)

Tips

- If you don't love heat, skip the chillies (or add another if you like it hot)!
- Not a fan of smoky flavour? Swap smoked paprika for sweet.
- You can buy passata, which is simply tomato and garlic, from any supermarket. It's a fantastic pantry staple. If you don't have passata handy, simply use 1 cup of fresh chopped tomatoes or a tin of chopped tomatoes instead.

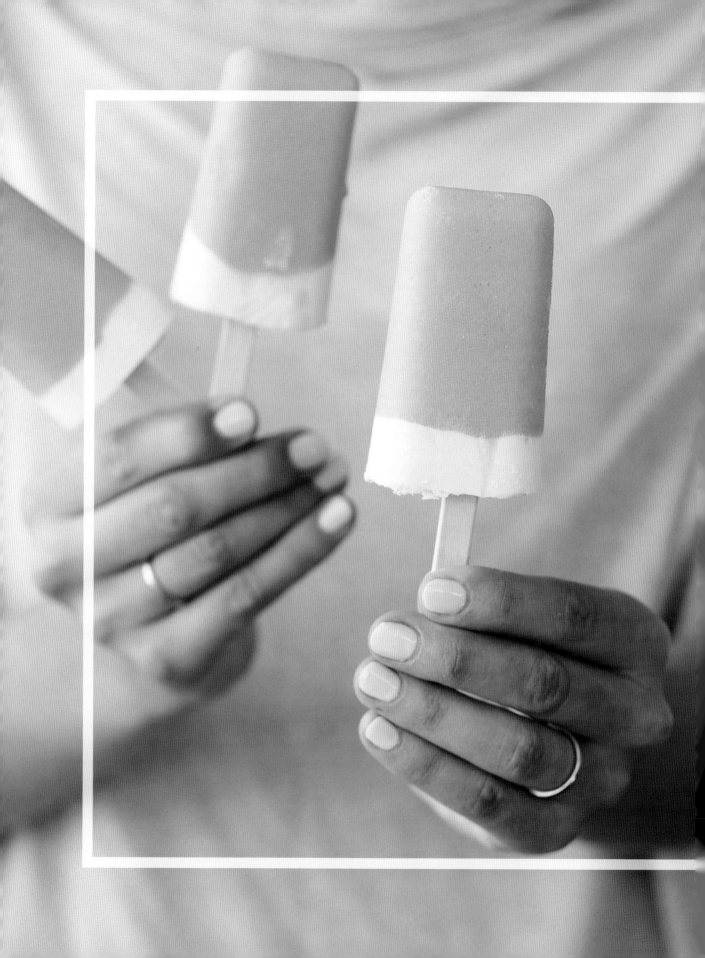

desserts

Not only will these cookies make your house smell fab, but you'll also be mistaken for a domestic superstar, even though they only contain four everyday ingredients. Kids will love helping you make these treats, as they couldn't be easier. Plus they're loaded with fibre and naturally nut- and gluten-free, making them a winner at the school bake sale.

Crazy like a coconut macaroons

PREP TIME: 5 MINUTES
COOKING TIME: 15–20 MINUTES

SERVES 12

2 ripe bananas
2 cups (130 g) shredded coconut
²/₃ cup (100 g) chocolate chips
A pinch of salt

Preheat the oven to 180°C (350°F). Line a baking tray with baking paper.

Mash the bananas in a bowl. Add the coconut, chocolate chips and salt and mix well. Scoop out about 1 heaped tablespoon of mixture per macaroon onto the baking tray. Press down lightly with a fork to flatten.

Bake for 15–20 minutes or until golden brown.

Tips

- *Play around with the recipe and try adding natural vanilla extract, cacao powder or cinnamon.*
- *You can also make this recipe into a coconut slice by spreading the mixture firmly onto a baking tray and cutting it into squares once it has cooled.*
- *Store in the fridge for up to a week (if they last that long).*
- *Use vegan-friendly chocolate chips if you are catering for vegans.*

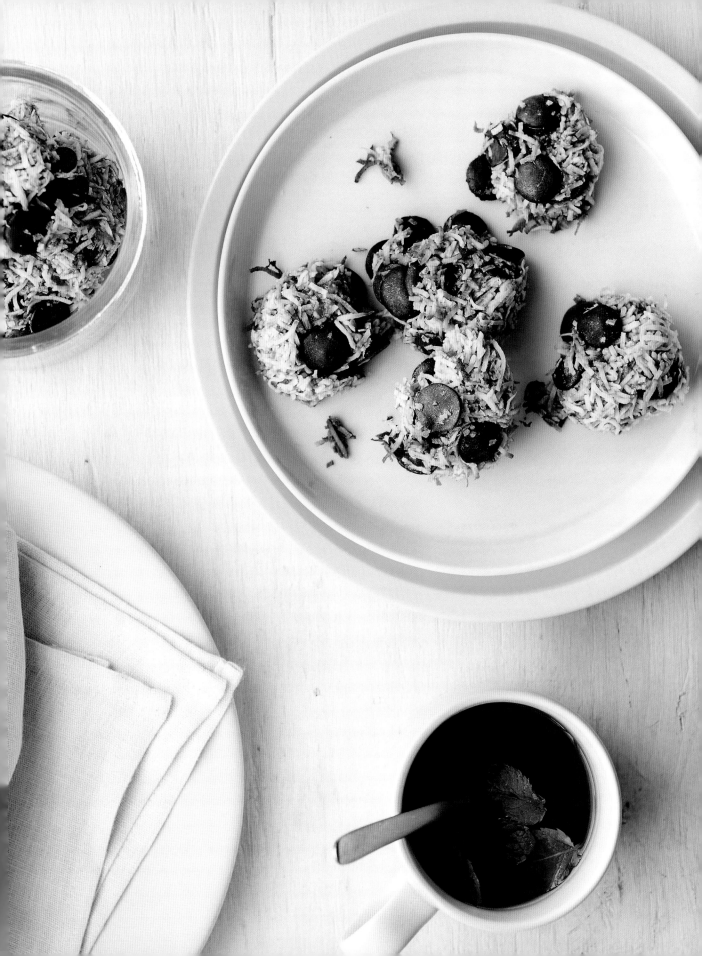

Chocolate mousse is my absolute favourite dessert. This five-ingredient recipe is light, fluffy and a much more nutritious version of the classic. Don't be alarmed that it uses something called aquafaba, which is the magical liquid you get from draining a tin of chickpeas. Trust me here: you won't even taste it. The end result is super-healthy, dead easy and mighty tasty.

Healthy chocolate mousse

PREP TIME: 5 MINUTES
COOKING TIME: 5 MINUTES
SETTING TIME: 15 MINUTES

SERVES 4

100 g (3½ oz) dark chocolate
   (at least 70% cocoa)
½ cup aquafaba (the liquid drained
   from a tin of chickpeas)
2 tablespoons pure maple syrup
1 teaspoon vanilla essence
   (optional)
A pinch of salt

Half-fill a small saucepan with water and heat over medium-low heat. Place a heatproof bowl on top, making sure the bottom of the bowl doesn't touch the water. Break in the chocolate pieces and stir occasionally until the chocolate has melted.

Meanwhile, put the aquafaba into the bowl of an electric mixer fitted with the whisk attachment. Whisk on high speed until the aquafaba forms stiff peaks. The aquafaba is ready when you can flip the bowl upside down and nothing falls out!

Carefully add the maple syrup, vanilla essence (if using) and salt and drizzle in the melted chocolate. Gently fold in the ingredients until just combined.

Pour the mixture into a serving bowl (or individual glasses) and transfer to the fridge to chill for at least 15 minutes before serving.

Tips

- *Use dairy-free chocolate to make this recipe vegan and dairy-free.*
- *Aquafaba is a fantastic alternative to eggs. I often use chickpeas in my cooking, so this recipe is a chance to use something that would have otherwise been thrown out. I find it works best when it's cold.*
- *Serve with shaved chocolate and fresh berries.*

No kidding, sticky date pudding would be my death-row meal (with pasta for mains). Not that I'm planning on doing anything crazy, but the thought has crossed my mind. This single-serve dessert is just perfect when you want a sweet treat in a jiffy. I love the rich flavour, chunky pieces of pecan and dates and the way I feel satisfied after eating this, especially when it's served with the better-for-you caramel sauce.

Stuck-in-the-mug sticky date pudding with caramel sauce

Put all of the cake ingredients in a small bowl and stir until well combined. Pour into a microwave-safe mug and cook for 90 seconds on High.

Meanwhile, mix together the ingredients for the caramel sauce. Pour onto the mug cake to serve.

Tips

- *Use gluten-free flour if you are sensitive.*
- *Replace the honey with maple syrup for a vegan version.*

PREP TIME: 3 MINUTES
COOKING TIME: 1½ MINUTES

SERVES 1

2 tablespoons self-raising flour
½ teaspoon ground cinnamon
½ banana, mashed
2 teaspoons extra virgin olive oil
1 teaspoon honey
6 pecans, chopped
2 fresh dates, pitted and chopped
A pinch of salt

CARAMEL SAUCE
1 teaspoon honey or maple syrup
2 teaspoons tahini
1 teaspoon water
A pinch of salt

Chocolate and peanut butter were made for each other. These delicious treats have far fewer ingredients than the ones you find at the supermarket.

Peanut butter pieces

PREP TIME: 5 MINUTES
COOKING TIME: 3 MINUTES
CHILLING TIME: 20 MINUTES

SERVES 10

1 cup (150 g) chopped dark
  chocolate
2 tablespoons milk
½ cup (140 g) 100% peanut butter
1 tablespoon maple syrup

Melt the chocolate in a microwave-safe bowl in 30-second bursts, stirring in the milk and a pinch of salt. Pour half the chocolate mixture into cupcake cases, tipping the chocolate along the sides to form a 'cup'. Freeze for 10 minutes to set the chocolate.

Meanwhile, mix the peanut butter with maple syrup and a pinch of salt. Scoop the peanut butter mixture into the chocolate cups, flattening the top. Finish by pouring the remaining chocolate on top, covering the peanut butter. Top with a sprinkle of salt and refrigerate for 10 minutes or until set.

Tips

- You'll need cupcake cases, or you can simply line a baking tray with baking paper and create a layered slab of goodness, from which you can cut delicious pieces of slice.
- Place the cupcake cases in a muffin tin to help them keep their shape.
- Use dairy-free or vegan chocolate and milk substitute if you like.

This dessert tastes like one of your favourite chocolate bars, with no compromise on flavour but way more of the wholesome stuff to enjoy. You'll be blown away by how easy it is to make, yet how good it tastes. This recipe is ideal to take along to friends for a tea, or when you're asked to bring nothing, but want to bring something.

Nutty chocolate slice

Line a baking tray with baking paper.

Put the pecans and dates into a food processor and blitz for 1–2 minutes or until it forms a crumb. Spread the crumbs on the prepared tray and press to flatten.

Mix the peanut butter and honey and spread it over the crumb layer.

Melt the chocolate in a microwave-proof bowl in 30-second bursts, stirring in the milk. Pour over the peanut butter layer. Sprinkle with salt flakes and freeze until set.

Cut into slices to serve.

PREP TIME: 10 MINUTES
COOKING TIME: 2 MINUTES

SERVES 15

110 g (3¾ oz) pecans
80 g (2¾ oz) dried pitted dates
½ cup (140 g) 100% peanut butter
3 tablespoons honey
100 g (3½ oz) dark chocolate
1 tablespoon milk
¼ teaspoon salt flakes

Tips

- *You can use fresh medjool dates if you like; about five medium pitted dates should do the trick.*
- *To make this dairy free and vegan, use nut milk, maple syrup instead of honey and make sure the chocolate is vegan friendly.*

I'll admit I'm not very good at baking. But this recipe is failproof: it's perfect each time I make it. This rich chocolate banana bread is my idea of a delicious treat, and a great way to use up overripe bananas! It's super-moist thanks to the Greek-style yoghurt and bananas so it won't dry up like ready-made varieties.

Chocolate banana bread

PREP TIME: 15 MINUTES
COOKING TIME: 45 MINUTES

SERVES 10–12

½ cup (50 g) rolled (porridge) oats

1 cup (150 g) plain flour

3 tablespoons cacao powder

1½ teaspoons bicarbonate of soda
  (baking soda)

7 fresh dates (or 14 dried dates,
  plus 1–2 tablespoons of water)

3 overripe bananas (about 1 cup
  mashed)

½ cup (65 g) Greek-style yoghurt

⅓ cup (80 ml) maple syrup

¼ teaspoon salt

2 large eggs

½ cup (85 g) chocolate chips
  (optional)

Preheat the oven to 175°C (345°F). Lightly grease a 13 x 23 cm (5 x 9 inch) loaf tin and set aside.

Blitz the oats in a food processor for 30 seconds or until rough flour.

In a large bowl, combine the plain flour, oats, cacao powder and bicarbonate of soda. Stir until well combined.

Put the dates in a food processor and blitz to a smooth paste. Add the bananas, yoghurt, maple syrup and salt and blitz for 10 seconds or until combined.

Lightly whisk the eggs in a medium bowl. Add the date mixture and stir to combine.

Pour the date mixture into the bowl with the flour mixture and add the chocolate chips, if using. Stir gently, but don't overmix.

Pour the batter into the prepared tin. Spread the mix evenly and bake for 40–45 minutes.

Cool in the tin for 10 minutes before turning the loaf onto a wire rack to cool completely.

Tips

- *If you have oat flour, use it instead of the rolled oats.*
- *The loaf will stay fresh and moist for 3–4 days after you've baked it. As it's just the two of us at home, I like to slice up the loaf and freeze the pieces individually.*

desserts

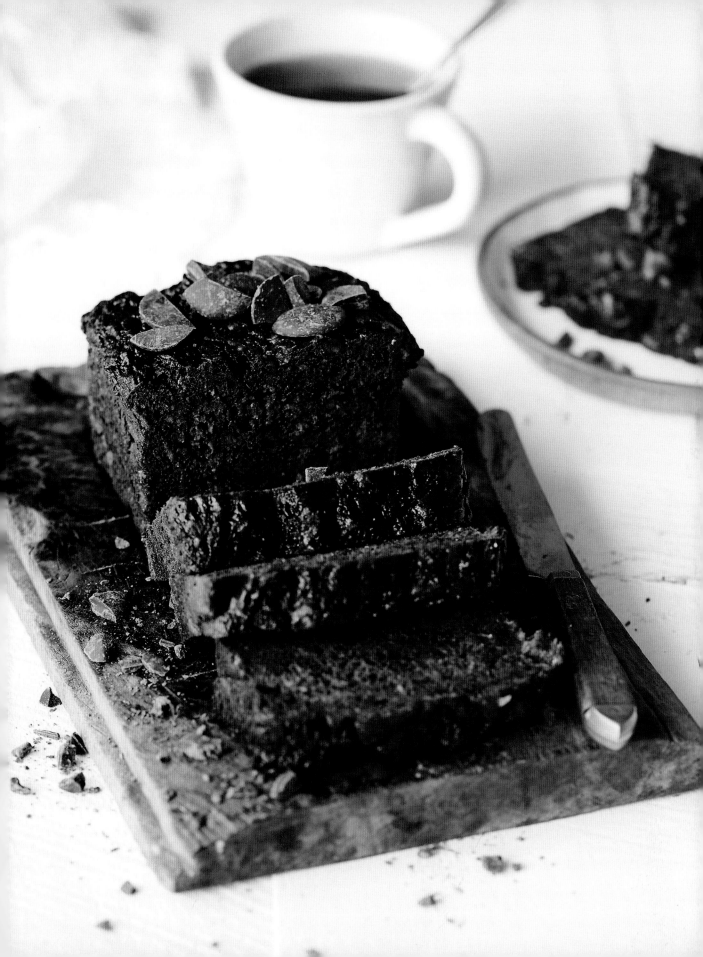

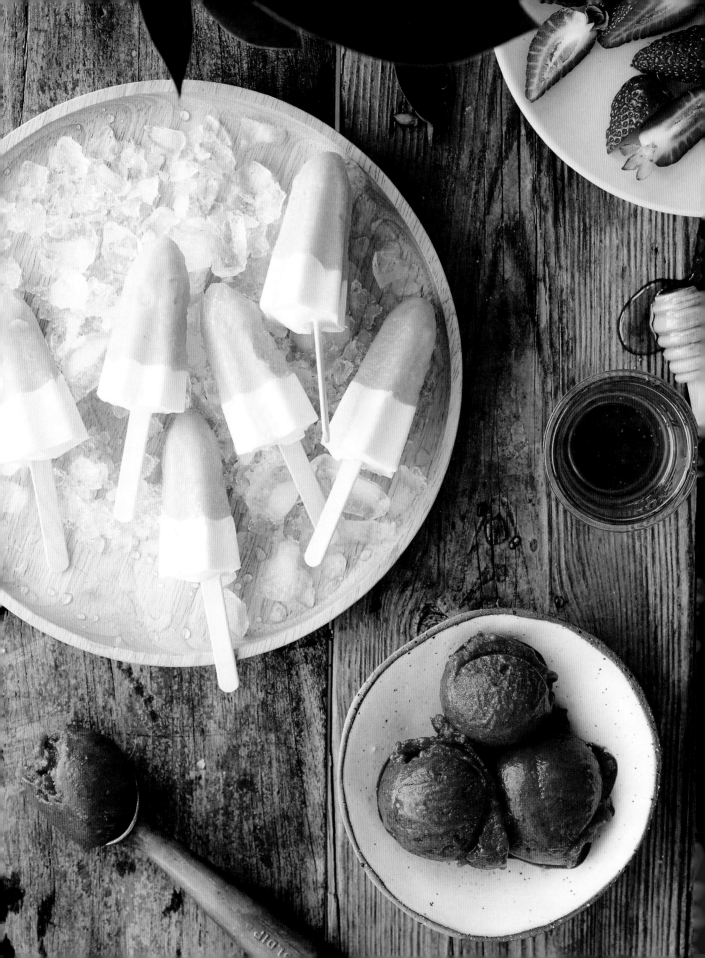

everyday option • gluten free • dairy free • vegan • low gi • high fibre
heart healthy • healthy ageing • diabetes friendly • nut free

I am obsessed with this simple, one-ingredient mango sorbet. When it's hot outside, you can bet I'm snacking on this. I almost feel silly writing this up as a 'recipe' because it's that easy but I wouldn't want you to miss out! I buy a tray of 'imperfect' mangoes and freeze the flesh ready to use.

Mango sorbet

Cut off the cheeks of the mango, then use the inside of a glass to scoop the flesh from the skin. Freeze for 2–3 hours until frozen.

Process the frozen mango in a food processor for 1–2 minutes or until it reaches soft ice-cream texture.

PREP TIME: 5 MINUTES
FREEZING TIME: 2–3 HOURS

SERVES 1

1 mango

I have a major sweet tooth and this sweet-and-sour strawberry sorbet really hits the spot. With only two ingredients, this healthy recipe will be ready in less than 5 minutes. This recipe is so refreshing, light and tasty. You're gonna love how easy it is! It's a fantastic healthy snack for kids and they will love seeing how it's made. You can also make this recipe with mixed berries.

Strawberry sorbet

Blitz both ingredients in a food processor for 1–2 minutes or until it becomes smooth sorbet texture. It will go powdery at first, so keep processing until it's smooth and creamy.

PREP TIME: 2 MINUTES

SERVES 2

250 g (9 oz) frozen strawberries
1 tablespoon honey or maple syrup

Got a killer craving for something sweet, but not much sweet stuff in the house? My go-to is often this simple banana nice cream. I freeze all overripe bananas for this exact purpose. It's a quick dessert to whip up, literally!

Banana nice cream

PREP TIME: 5 MINUTES

SERVES 2

80 g (2¾ oz) raw almonds

2 frozen bananas

1 cup ice cubes

2 tablespoons 100% nut butter

3 teaspoons cacao powder
   (optional)

Process the almonds in a food processor to fine crumbs. Add the remaining ingredients with a pinch of salt and blend until smooth.

Tips

- *You can use whatever nuts you have available, so play around with it.*
- *Add the cacao powder to turn this into chocolate nice cream.*
- *Use this as a base recipe and play around by adding your favourite ingredients, such as coconut or vanilla, or top it with granola.*

This is a healthier, less-processed version of one of my favourite summertime ice treats. It's perfect for balmy summer nights as an after-dinner treat. Kids will love this beauty of a recipe.

Mango ice-cream bars

Peel the mangoes and put the flesh in a food processor. Blitz until smooth. Spoon the mixture into the bottom of 12 popsicle moulds and transfer to the freezer for at least 1 hour.

Mix the cream and maple syrup together, then pour on top of the mango in the popsicle molds, leaving a little space at the top of each mould to allow the liquid to expand. Insert the sticks. Freeze for 2 hours before unmoulding to serve.

PREP TIME: 10 MINUTES
FREEZING TIME: 3 HOURS

SERVES 12

2 ripe mangoes
300 ml (10½ fl oz) thickened (whipping) cream
1 tablespoon maple syrup

Tips

- It's a great way to use up ripe mangoes (once you've bought the whole tray).
- You'll need 12 popsicle molds for this recipe. They are available from supermarkets and homeware stores. You could also use styrofoam cups and food-grade popsicle sticks or a plastic spoon for the handle.
- Don't eat dairy? Use coconut cream instead.

These no-bake brownies are seriously simple – and I've got a feeling
you're going to love them as much as I do. If I have a craving after dinner,
I'll sometimes whip up a batch of these.

Salted peanut butter chocolate 'brownies'

PREP: 10 MINUTES

MAKES 8–10

²/₃ cup (100 g) almonds, skin on

3 tablespoons peanut butter

3 tablespoons cacao powder

½ cup (80 g) dried dates, pitted

¼ teaspoon salt

Line a baking tray with baking paper. Combine all of the
ingredients in a food processor and blitz until it becomes
a rough dough. if you squeeze it together and it sticks,
it's ready. If not, process a little longer.

Pour the mixture into the prepared tray, pressing down
to compress.

Eat straight away or refrigerate. Cut into 5 cm (2 inch)
squares to serve.

Tips

- You can store the 'brownies' in the fridge in
  an airtight container for 1 week or freeze
  them to keep fresh for longer.
- Roll the mixture into balls instead for
  delicious energy balls you can pack and
  carry for a sweet treat.

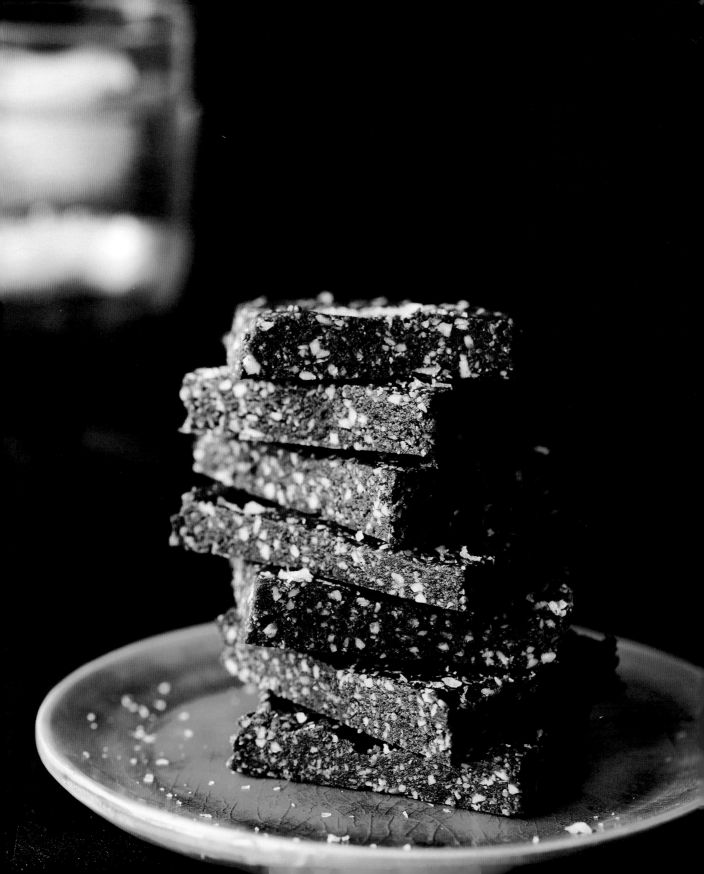

INDEX

adrenaline, 121
affirmations, 115
alcohol, 120, 137
amino acids, 51
anxiety, 90, 120, 124, 125
appetite, 21, 22, 26
artificial sweeteners, 49

balanced eating, 34–35
balanced meal guide, 72–73
batch cooking, 66–67
beauty, 57–58
binge eating, 8, 78–79, 80, 89, 103
binge-eating disorder, 103
bliss balls, 51
blood glucose, 46–47
body bullies, 107–109
body dysmorphia, 100–101
body, healthy, 109–110
body image, 58, 100–115, 109–110, 113
body love touch, 114
body mass index (BMI), 57, 64
boredom, 90
boundaries, 132
bullies, body, 107–109
busyness, 133

canned food, 42
carbohydrates, 40, 46–47, 70, 73
chemicals, 118–119
children, teaching, 97
clean eating, 15, 35
coconut oil, 53
coconut sugar, 48
coffee, 53
comfort foods, 22
comparisons, 104
convenience health foods, 67
cortisol, 121
counsellor, 90, 103
cravings, 49, 79, 80, 92
'crowding', 30, 39

dairy foods, 52
depression, 125
dieting, 7–10, 14–17, 58–59, 80
dried fruit, 43
dysmorphia, body, 100–101

eating disorders, 100–103
eating habits, 31, 62
emails, 135
emotional eating, 8, 78–82, 89, 92, 94
energy, 118–119
everyday foods, 84
exercise, 7, 119, 122, 124, 126–131

fat, 52–53, 70, 73, 118
fibre, 48, 119
food police, 107–109
food, relationship with, 78–97
forbidden foods, 80, 84, 85, 89
forgiveness, 112
fridge, healthy, 65, 143
frozen food, 42, 66
fructose, 43
fruit, 30, 42–43, 70
fruit juice, 43

ghrelin, 121
Glycemic Index (GI), 46–47
grief, 103
grocery shopping, 65
guilt, 92–95

habits, 49, 62, 64–65, 82, 120
healthy diet, 64, 125
healthy weight, 56, 64
herb garden, 66
hormones, 23, 49, 92, 118–21
hunger, 21–31, 65, 80, 81
hunger diary, 28, 30–31
hunger scale, 22–23

insulin, 121
intuitive eating, 20–31

judgement, 90, 105–107, 112

#keepitreal, 56, 64
kitchen, healthy, 65

language, food, 82
leptin, 23, 121

maple syrup, 48
meal prepping, 66–67
Mediterranean-style eating, 34
mental health, 125
mindset, 56, 103
moderation, 34–35
mood, 118–120, 124–125

negative self talk, 115
nuts, 70, 89

obesity, 56
oestrogen, 121
oil, 53, 70
omega-3 fatty acids, 53
omega-6 fatty acids, 53
organic food, 42
orthorexia, 101
overeating, 23, 94–95
overexercising, 129
overweight, 56

pantry, healthy, 65, 142
perfectionism, 110
phyto-oestrogens, 119
police, food, 107–109
portion sizes, 70
probiotics, 119
protein, 51, 70, 73
protein balls, 51
protein powders, 52
psychologist, 90, 103

relationship with food, 78–97
relationships, 135
restrictive diets, 14
rice malt syrup, 48
rituals, 120
routine, 120, 122

RECIPE INDEX

salads, 38
scarcity mindset, 87, 103
self-acceptance, 110–112
self-care, 131, 133
self-compassion, 110
self-control, 80
self-sabotage, 105
self talk, negative, 115
serotonin, 121
shopping, 65
skin, 138–139
sleep, 49, 90, 118, 122, 136–137
snacks, healthy, 30, 69–70
social media, 90, 104, 113, 135
sometimes foods, 84
starchy vegetables, 40
stevia, 49
stress, 90, 120, 124
sugar, 48–49
superfoods, 35–36
supermarkets, 65
sweeteners, 49

technology, 135
testosterone, 121
thyroid hormones, 121
trauma, 103
TV, 81, 90

underweight, 56

vegetables, 30, 37–42, 70, 73

waste, reducing, 75
weekends, 91
weigh-ins, 7, 64
weight loss, 7–10, 14–15, 56–59, 90, 107
weight range, 56
weight stigma, 57
wholefoods, 37, 119
willpower, 80–81

asparagus: Maple-chilli sauté greens, 204
avocado
    Avocado dressing, 179
    Holy moly chunky guacamole!, 208

Baked pumpkin with feta, 198
balsamic dressing, Basic, 205
bananas
    Banana nice cream, 224
    Chocolate banana bread, 220
Basic balsamic dressing, 205
beans
    Nonna's minestrone, 175
    Quinoa burrito bowl in the slow cooker, 182
beef
    Mumma's meatballs, 170
    Vegie-full beef bolognese with real spaghetti, 166
Berry good breakfast bowl, 156
Big breakfast bowl, 146
bolognese with real spaghetti, Vegie-full beef, 166
'brownies', Salted peanut butter chocolate, 226

Caesar salad with creamy avocado dressing, 179
Caramel sauce, 217
Cheater's chicken slaw, 184
Cheeky tzatziki, 210
chia pudding, Chocolate, 149
chicken
    Cheater's chicken slaw, 184
    Green chicken stir-fry, 178
    Quinoa burrito bowl in the slow cooker, 182
    Twenty-minute tacos, 188
    Zucchini noodle pad Thai, 172
chickpeas
    Loaded Greek salad, two ways, 197
    Mediterranean lunch bowl, 196
    Pumpkin falafel, 187
Chilli garlic snow peas, 201
chocolate
    Chocolate banana bread, 220
    Chocolate chia pudding, 149
    Crazy like a coconut macaroons, 214
    Healthy chocolate mousse, 216

    Natural chocolate protein bar, 162
    Nutty chocolate slice, 219
    Peanut butter pieces, 218
    Salted peanut butter chocolate 'brownies', 226
coconut macaroons, 214
corn: Quinoa burrito bowl in the slow cooker, 182
Crazy like a coconut macaroons, 214

date pudding with caramel sauce, Stuck-in-the-mug sticky, 217
dips
    Cheeky tzatziki, 210
    Holy moly chunky guacamole!, 208
dressings, 184, 197, 205
    Avocado dressing, 179
    Basic balsamic dressing, 205
    Honey lime dressing, 195
    Poke bowl dressing, 205
    Tahini dressing, 205
    Zesty dressing, 206

Easy like a Sunday morning eggs, 161
Eat the rainbow grated salad, 206
eggs
    Big breakfast bowl, 146
    Easy like a Sunday morning eggs, 161
Energy-boosting green smoothie, 150

falafel, Pumpkin, 187
Family favourite flatbread pizzas, 169
feta, Baked pumpkin with, 198
fish
    Maple soy sriracha one-tray salmon, 176
    Mediterranean lunch bowl, 196
    Seedy crumbed fish, 185
    Sesame-crusted fish, 181
    Terrifically tasty teriyaki salmon, 171
freekeh salad, Freeken' good, 195
Freeken' good freekeh salad, 195

Garlicky parmesan mushrooms, 203
Get-up-and-go overnight oats, 155
Goldilocks' favourite power porridge, 158
Greek salad, two ways, Loaded, 197
Green chicken stir-fry, 178
guacamole!, Holy moly chunky, 208

Hail Caesar salad with creamy avocado dressing, 179
Healthy chocolate mousse, 216
Holy moly chunky guacamole!, 208
Honey lime dressing, 195

ice cream
    Banana nice cream, 224
    Mango ice-cream bars, 225

juice, Post-bender booster green, 159

lamb: Mumma's meatballs, 170
Les's spicy tomato sauce, 211
Lifesaving baked rainbow vegetables, 200
Loaded Greek salad, two ways, 197
Lyndi's healthy home-made muesli, 152

macaroons, Crazy like a coconut, 214
mango
    Mango ice-cream bars, 225
    Mango sorbet, 223
Maple-chilli sauté greens, 204
Maple soy sriracha one-tray salmon, 176
meatballs, Mumma's, 170
Mediterranean lunch bowl, 196
minestrone, Nonna's, 175
mousse, Healthy chocolate, 216
muesli, Lyndi's healthy home-made, 152
Mumma's meatballs, 170
mushrooms, Garlicky parmesan, 203

Natural chocolate protein bar, 162
Nonna's minestrone, 175
Nutty chocolate slice, 219

oats
    Berry good breakfast bowl, 156
    Get-up-and-go overnight oats, 155
    Goldilocks' favourite power porridge, 158
    Lyndi's healthy home-made muesli, 152

pad Thai, Zucchini noodle, 172
pantry essentials, 142
pasta: Vegie-full beef bolognese with real spaghetti, 166
peanut butter
    Peanut butter pieces, 218
    Salted peanut butter chocolate 'brownies', 226
peanut sauce, 209
pizzas, flatbread, 169
Poke bowl dressing, 205
pomegranate tabouleh, Quinoa, 192
porridge, 158
Post-bender booster green juice, 159
Pretty perfect peanut sauce, 209
protein bar, Natural chocolate, 162
pudding with caramel sauce, Stuck-in-the-mug sticky date, 217
pudding, Chocolate chia, 149
pumpkin
    Baked pumpkin with feta, 198
    Pumpkin falafel, 187

quinoa
    Quinoa burrito bowl in the slow cooker, 182
    Quinoa pomegranate tabouleh, 192

salads
    Baked pumpkin with feta, 198
    Cheater's chicken slaw, 184
    Eat the rainbow grated salad, 206
    Freeken' good freekeh salad, 195
    Hail Caesar salad with creamy avocado dressing, 179
    Lifesaving baked rainbow vegetables, 200
    Loaded Greek salad, two ways, 197
    Mediterranean lunch bowl, 196
    Quinoa pomegranate tabouleh, 192

salmon
    Maple soy sriracha one-tray salmon, 176
    Terrifically tasty teriyaki salmon, 171
Salted peanut butter chocolate 'brownies', 226
Seedy crumbed fish, 185
Sesame-crusted fish, 181
slice, Nutty chocolate, 219
slow cooker, Quinoa burrito bowl in the, 182
smoothie, Energy-boosting green, 150
snow peas, Chilli garlic, 201
sorbets
    Mango sorbet, 223
    Strawberry sorbet, 223
soup: Nonna's minestrone, 175
spaghetti, Vegie-full beef bolognese with real, 166
sticky date pudding with caramel sauce, Stuck-in-the-mug, 217
stir-fry, Green chicken, 178
Strawberry sorbet, 223
Stuck-in-the-mug sticky date pudding with caramel sauce, 217

tabouleh, Quinoa pomegranate, 192
tacos, Twenty-minute, 188
Tahini dressing, 205
Terrifically tasty teriyaki salmon, 171
toast, four ways, 153
tomatoes
    Easy like a Sunday morning eggs, 161
    Les's spicy tomato sauce, 211
    Nonna's minestrone, 175
tuna: Mediterranean lunch bowl, 196
Twenty-minute tacos, 188
tzatziki, Cheeky, 210

Vegie-full beef bolognese with real spaghetti, 166

Zesty dressing, 206
Zucchini noodle pad Thai, 172

REFERENCES

CHAPTER 3

1 Daniel Borota, Elizabeth Murray, Gizem Keceli, Allen Chang, Joseph M Watabe, Maria Ly, John P Toscano & Michael A Yassa, Post-study caffeine administration enhances memory consolidation in humans, *Nature Neuroscience* volume 17, pages 201–203 (2014), doi:10.1038/nn.3623

2 Bravi, Francesca et al. Coffee reduces risk for hepatocellular carcinoma: an updated meta-analysis, *Clinical Gastroenterology and Hepatology* Volume 11, Issue 11, 1413–1421.e1

CHAPTER 4

1 Afzal S, Tybjærg-Hansen A, Jensen GB, Nordestgaard BG. Change in Body Mass Index associated with lowest mortality in Denmark, 1976–2013. *JAMA*. 2016;315(18):1989–1996. doi:10.1001/jama.2016.4666

2 Waaler, H.T., 1984: Height, weight and mortality. The Norwegian experience. *Acta Medica Scandinavica* (Suppl. 679): 56

3 Flegal KM1, Graubard BI, Williamson DF, Gail MH. Excess deaths associated with underweight, overweight, and obesity. *JAMA*. 2005 Apr 20;293(15):1861–7.

4 Marina Garas, D.O.; Mary B. Roberts, M.S.; Molly E. Waring, Ph.D.; Christine M. Albert, M.D., M.P.H.; Deepika Laddu, Ph.D.; Marcia L Stefanick, Ph.D.; David K. Garas, M.B.A.; and Charles B. Eaton, M.D., M.S. Yo-yo dieting dangerous even if you're not overweight American Heart Association Meeting Report – Poster: T2041 – Session: LF.APS.P226

CHAPTER 5

1 Muraven M, Baumeister RF, Self-regulation and depletion of limited resources: does self-control resemble a muscle? *Psychological Bulletin*, 2000 Mar; 126(2):247–59.

2 Pesch, Megan H. et al. Mothers of obese children use more direct imperatives to restrict eating. *Journal of Nutrition Education and Behavior*, Volume 50, Issue 4, 403–407.e1

CHAPTER 6

1 eatingdisorders.org.au/key-research-a-statistics

CHAPTER 7

1 BPA is bisphenol A, a synthetic compound found in some plastics that can leach into food. It's an oestrogen imitator and research is ongoing into its possible effects on humans. To be on the safe side, avoid it if you can.

2 T3 and T4 are the short names for the tyrosine-based hormones produced in the thyroid gland. They are triiodothyronine (T3) and thyroxine (T4).

ACKNOWLEDGMENTS

An incredibly big thank you to everyone who helped make this book possible.

Firstly, a massive thank you to my followers and wonderful community. I've got the most-lovely humans joining me online to share our experiences and recipes and ideas.

To all the nutritionists and dietitians who spread messages of balance: keep doing your work. We need your voices to help clear through the clutter.

Thank you to Jane, Melody, Madeleine, Kelly, Carol, Britta and Jemma – and all the incredibly talented people who make Murdoch Books so truly wonderful.

To my Sydney community, who helped raise me, and the friends I've made along the way, from school and university. Thank you for being so loyal and supportive.

A massive thank you to my amazing and incredible family – the Polivnicks, Cohens, Conradies and Koltais – for playing such a big role in my life. (And for letting me photograph the food at Shabbat dinner before you get to eat any of it!)

For my late Bobba, Sonia, for teaching me a love of food; for my late Ouma, Louise, for passing on to me a lust for life; and my Oupa, Frans, for teaching me the importance of a good joke.

For my brothers, Ryan and Warren, thanks for making me robust and tougher than I ever thought I was, for 'being in my blog', and for sometimes letting me play with you when we were young.

I can't thank my parents, Elize and Dennis Polivnick, enough for your constant love, for giving me the world and for being my biggest supporters.

And a special thank you to my husband, Les, for enthusiastically testing all new recipes with me, even the ones that didn't work out, and most importantly for being my ultimate partner and friend.

Published in 2019 by Murdoch Books,
an imprint of Allen & Unwin

Murdoch Books Australia
83 Alexander Street,
Crows Nest NSW 2065
Phone: +61 (0)2 8425 0100
murdochbooks.com.au
info@murdochbooks.com.au

Murdoch Books UK
Ormond House,
26–27 Boswell Street,
London, WC1N 3JZ
Phone: +44 (0) 20 8785 5995
murdochbooks.co.uk
info@murdochbooks.co.uk

For Corporate Orders & Custom Publishing
contact our business development team at
salesenquiries@murdochbooks.com.au

Publisher: Kelly Doust
Editorial Manager: Jane Price
Editor: Melody Lord
Design Manager: Madeleine Kane
Design Concept: Fleur Anson
Designer: Hugh Ford
Illustrations: Estee Sarsfield
Photography: Cath Muscat, Leah Stanistreet
and Luca Prodigo
Stylist: Sarah O'Brien
Food preparation at shoot: Ross Dobson
Production Director: Lou Playfair

ISBN 978 1 76052 374 9 Australia
ISBN 978 1 91163 200 9 UK

A cataloguing-in-publication entry is available
from the catalogue of the National Library of
Australia at nla.gov.au
A catalogue record for this book is available
from the British Library

Colour reproduction by Splitting Image Colour
Studio Pty Ltd, Clayton, Victoria
Printed by 1010 Printing Co Ltd, China

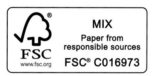

MIX
Paper from
responsible sources
FSC® C016973
FSC
www.fsc.org

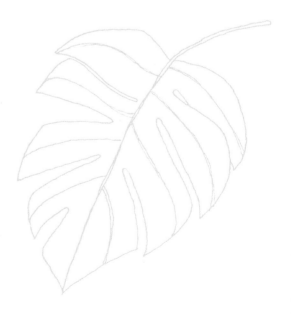